SOS: Switch Off Stress

I0439190

A First Aid Kit

101 practical techniques for stopping distress
in 6 seconds to 6 minutes

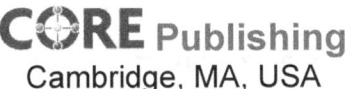 **Publishing**
Cambridge, MA, USA

Print version of SOS © 2014 by Sharon Seivert

Images: Cover photo is by Rafi, GraphicsFuel.com; license is royalty-free for personal and commercial use. Sharon Seivert owns all logo images, *The Balancing Act* book cover, and personal photos. Photos in Chapters 1-4 are licensed from *Dreamstime*; Chapter 5 photo is by Judy Selednik; Chapter 6 photo is from NASA. Color images for this black & white book can be seen at www.thecoreporation.com/sos_links.

THIS SOS "FIRST AID KIT" WILL HELP YOU:

Get immediate relief from the pain of distress…

…in only 6 seconds to 6 minutes.

Protect your health with these fast, effective responses.

Switch Off a reactive stress response (_Fight/Flight_) and…

…_Switch On_ a proactive one (_Find/Flourish_ or _Learn/Thrive_).

Transform Stress from an Enemy into a Teacher/Friend.

Cope more effectively with the everyday challenges of stress.

Make new habits from your favorite SOS techniques.

Discover valuable resources where you can learn more.

Take a micro-vacation every day.

Pass on SOS tools to adults and children you love so they…

…avoid toxic stress, protect themselves, and thrive.

TESTIMONIALS

Switch Off Stress offers very practical ways to deal with acute anxiety and intimidating situations. As a physician, I recommend this book to my fellow physicians and to patients who are looking for a non-medication way to handle current stress and gain long-term benefits. (I have observed highly stressed men in re-entry programs benefit from SOS "games", which made them laugh and kept them out of harms way.)

- Arlene Reed-Delaney, M.D. (Psychiatrist)

Many years ago I used to get upset every time I got stuck in heavy traffic in São Paulo, my hometown. Then I started listening to audiobooks while commuting, a pleasant habit I've kept up since then. Thus, the 'enemy' became my ally. SOS: Switch Off Stress is a blueprint for making stress your friend. It is packed with an amazing array of tested, practical, valuable techniques. Sharon Seivert promises to help you relieve stress in 6 seconds to 6 minutes, but these teachings will stick with you long after you've put the book down. As an avid reader of Sharon's work, I have read, applied - and loved - her latest book. Sharon, you did splendidly again!

- Paulo Rovai, Marketing Executive, Toyota/Lexus Brazil

SOS: Switch Off Stress provides many easy and effective tools people need to quickly overcome stress, calm down and get centered. _This book is a MASTERPIECE_…a breath of fresh air (like you've given me permission to breathe). The freedom this book will provide to those who use it is astonishing. SOS is brilliant—a must read for all! Thank you for your amazing work, beautiful heart and passion to help so many.

— Andrea Kazanjian, CMO and SVP, Travel Hopscotch

Sharon Seivert is a genius! Switch Off Stress _shows her special understanding of the often-hidden anxieties of modern day high achievers. In this well researched, must-have book she_ provides _a healthy dose of practical advice and wit to help readers resolve real, everyday weighty concerns. Problem solving has never been addressed in a better way."_

- Kevin Armstrong, General Counsel
DST Brokerage Solutions, LLC

Sharon Seivert has written an incredibly generous book; this is THE go-to book to help all of us in our accelerated lives. Drawing from a wide-range of traditions and practices, she has distilled what could be complex material into extremely useful daily practices that WILL keep us centered. Thank you, Sharon!

- Moe Ross, CEO/Founder, Miographies

SOS can be used in the moment to reduce stress and over time as a toolkit for living life to the fullest. With such a variety

4

of techniques all in one place, you can turn to any page and find something that hits the spot. I know I will be going back to this fantastic resource time and time again.

-   Louisa Mattson, Ph.D., Psychologist & Career Consultant

Switch Off Stress *is a must-have for every entrepreneur's toolkit. It's brim-full with practical stress-reducing techniques. We recommend that entrepreneurs get this book, read it carefully, and then choose their own top 10 best techniques. Switching off Stress is key to finding, and staying on, the fast track to growing a young business.*

-   Dan Loague & Randy Reade,
    President & EVP, Washington D.C. ArchAngels

Sharon changed my life! She coached me to manage my stress while I changed careers several years ago. Not only did I get the job I wanted, in the new industry I wanted, and at a fantastic hospital—she helped me create a much happier, balanced and healthy lifestyle that has lasted to this day. Now Sharon has gathered many of the stress reduction techniques that helped me through those tough times and put them into a gift basket for others. I enthusiastically recommend SOS.

-   Chantal Stephens, Director of Marketing, Orlando Health

SOS: Switch Off Stress *is like having your own emotional emergency room at your fingertips—rapid techniques for relief when you need it, right now, and deeper insight to help you stay well the rest of the time.*

— Frederick Reed, President, ThoughtSigns

It was one of those mornings I felt drained. My to-do-list was too long and I could not decide what to do first. I picked up the SOS book to find out how to make stress my friend. After a quick glance at the introduction, I started work on my Mission. Within a minute of doing one technique, my fear had turned into faith, my frustration into energy and inspiration. Wow! That day I came up with the wonderful idea of integrating SOS into my "I Learn to Learn" training for high school students.

- Tamar van der Meer, Coach and Trainer, Netherlands

Sharon, your words always brought me inspiration and strength when I needed it the most. This guide will be a handy reference to use when you aren't around. For this, I thank you.

- Steve Oneto, Q.A. Manager, Walt Disney Company

SOS helped me right away. I started using the SING THOSE BLUES AWAY technique, and immediately got so much energy back that I was able to finish work that had been on my mind for days. I also experienced a full night of sleep, which I have not had in weeks, after watching the SOS sleep videos. *I feel that SOS made me stop—and brought me back to myself.*

- Cristina Gomez Castellano, Owner, TrendMarketIn

Here is *a convenient, easy way to chase the blues of stress away*. *Sharon's book* Switch Off Stress *is the First Aid Kit to save the day. I will recommend it to my clients.*

- Malik Rashid, Mental Health Counselor/Clinician

I've been searching for a resource to share with my life coaching and yoga clients that would encourage them to become the CEO's of their lives and "fire" their stressors by utilizing short sound bytes techniques. Sharon's new book is my answer—it's like having a personal Board of (stress-busting) Directors at your fingertips!

- Maripat Abbott, Founder of HolisticRelo.com

I love the light and joyful way you have written this book! SOS is a cheerful way to get rid of stress and feel more centered. And you make it so easy for coaches to work with this material! I will practice an exercise with my client during a session &/or give an activity as homework. It is so good that clients can actually FEEL the energy of each Balancing Act element.

- Laura Alders, Personal Coach, Netherlands

I've discovered that SOS is a <u>wonderful book for teachers</u> to use for quick techniques to help students focus their energy on class work. It's also a terrific resource for educators who need to relax and refresh after a long workday.

> \- Dorothy A. Ginnett, Ph.D.
> High School and College Science Teacher

Sharon Seivert's impressive book SOS: Switch Off Stress *is a very readable compendium of time-honored stress management approaches from diverse cultural origins. While people often habitually rely on a small cadre of stress control techniques, Sharon's book <u>gracefully opens the door to a plethora of ways to limit stress, restore inner balance, and renew one's vigor. This book is practical, inspirational, and enjoyable</u>. I strongly recommend it!*

> \- Steven Cavaleri, Ph.D., Professor of Management,
> Central Connecticut State University

TABLE OF CONTENTS

TABLE OF TIMING:
6 Seconds to 6 Minutes

Chapter One: Strengthen Your Core (SOS #1—#17)

<6 to 120 seconds: Emergency Breath; Breathe a Smile In—Breathe Toxins Out; No More Waiting to Exhale; Call a Time-out; Make Space around the Pain.
2 to 4 minutes: Stealth Breath; Countdown; Sing those Blues Away; Beam Me Up; Lightning Strikes; Sounds and Silence.
4 to 6 minutes: Experience the Calming Core Element; Walking Breath; Soothing Sounds; Small Universe; Access Your GPS; Talk to Your Smartest Self.

Chapter Two: Soothe Your Mind (SOS #18—#34)

<6 to 120 seconds: Stop It; Slow Down your Brain Waves; Give Your Eyes a Break; Participant/Observer Dual Lens; Reframe Stress as a Friend and Teacher.
2 to 4 minutes: Take a Laughter Break; The Tetris Effect; Get Inspired; Time Travel: Anticipation & Memories; C'mon, Get Happy; How Did You Contribute to This?
4 to 6 minutes: Experience the Inspiring Vision Element; How Much Will this Matter in…?; Mental Shielding; Mirror of the Mind; Subliminal Stress Relief; Stop It! (v2); Observe, Ask, Learn, Adapt.

Chapter Three: Blast Through Obstacles (SOS #35—#51)

<6 to 120 seconds: Set a Strong Intention; Just Do It; Activate Your Energy (The 20-second Rule); Stand Up; Power Poses.
2 to 4 minutes: Experience the Motivating Element of Mission; Do One Thing; Shake it, Baby, Shake it!; Now Power; Never Fail; Respect Your Desires; Reduce Resistance.
4 to 6 minutes: 5 Rites of Rejuvenation; Dance; Short Bursts; Change, Accept or Leave; Choose Your Weapon (Conflict Style).

Chapter Four: Improve Emotional Intelligence (#52—#68)

<6 to 120 seconds: Small Acts of Kindness; Smile; Give (and Get) a Hug; Say Thank You; Loving Kindness (short version); Smile at Three Extra People; Reversal Tapping; What are You Feeling?
2 to 4 minutes: Get Over Yourself; Tend and Befriend; Loving Kindness; Green--Yellow--Red Light; Connect with a Critter.
4 to 6 minutes: Experience Compassionate Element of Interactions; Transform Negative Emotions (EFT); Percussive Suggestion Technique (PSTEC); Find a Choir to Join; Try Laughter Yoga.

Chapter Five: Build Healthier Habits (SOS #69—#85)

<6 to 120 seconds: Ear Massage; Hydrate Your Body; Bless What You Eat and Drink; Remind Yourself to Eat Slowly; Get a Boost from Brain Food.
2 to 4 minutes: Experience the Steadying Element of Structure; Red Flag!; Eat an Apple a Day; Treat One of Your 5 Senses; Schedule Stress Breaks.
4 to 6 minutes: Show Me the Money; S-t-r-e-t-c-h; Brain Gym; Tea Time; You Snooze—You Win; Take a Break in Nature; Clean-Sort-Move-File.

Chapter Six: Experience Greater Ease (SOS #86—#101)

<6 to 120 seconds: Ho'oponopono; I Am That I Am; When in Doubt, Pray; All is Well; The 5 Element Mantra.
2 to 4 minutes: Experience the Flow of Synergy; Get a Great Night's Sleep (Top 10 Tricks); Express Gratitude; Find the Roots of Your Distress; Re-balance with the Balance Beam.
4 to 6 minutes: The Healing Code; OM Sounding; Healing Circle; Get the Binaural Beat; Portable Spa Treatment; This Too Will Pass (The Holographic Universe)

*Note: For direct links to instructions and other resources for the above SOS techniques, go to a special web page created just for this book: "**www.thecoreporation.com/sos_links**".*

BACKGROUND

I built this book for speed and ease of navigation. For this reason, **Section I** lists only the "first aid Instructions" for each *Switch Off Stress* technique so you can get immediate relief from the pain of distress—in only 6 seconds to 6 minutes.

In **Section II**, you'll find more information about each SOS activity so you have all the information you need to make a new habit out of any rapid-response tool you particularly like.

In **Section III: Appendices**, I've noted further details if you wish more information about the Background for SOS.

Special web resource addendum for this book: *SOS: Switch Off Stress* was originally designed as an *EvaBook* (electronic-video-audio book) with links that readers could click on to be taken directly to instructional aids. However, I had so many requests for a print version of SOS that I decided to respond. In order to approximate the *EvaBook* experience of getting stress relief within 6 seconds to 6 minutes, I created a special on-line resource (**www.*thecoreporation.com/sos_links*)** with all the direct instructional links mentioned in this print version of SOS. I suggest you bookmark this "sos_links" webpage in your computer or smartphone for ease and speed of use.

Additionally, you will find each URL reference listed in this print book so you can type that link in your browser, if you prefer to do so. (Prefixes are "http://youtube.com/watch?..." for videos and "http://www." for web sites, unless otherwise noted.)

A Personal Note, Dedication, and Thank You

As an integral part of my executive, leader, and career coaching, I teach clients how to use *The Balancing Act* to switch their stress into a teacher or friend who will help them create healthier and happier lives, relationships and work. In this process I have learned what keeps people stuck versus what breaks them out of dysfunctional patterns so they can respond more effectively to the challenges of stress, change for good, and thrive. And, since my policy is to recommend only what I've personally tried out myself, I have taken every opportunity to practice what I preach by testing many stress-busting activities.

Indeed, I wrote this book in part to help myself survive a long period of distress. As a result, I can state unequivocally that each one of these 101 techniques works very well, indeed. Today, at the end of what has been a long, winding, and very hard road, I am able to smile out from these pages. I am extraordinarily grateful to have emerged from these recent trials with strong health, a positive attitude, increased confidence, and a deeper faith in the beneficence of the universe. (If you're interested in learning about the personal challenges SOS helped me meet, go to Appendix A, Background.

In *SOS: Switch Off Stress* I am delighted to introduce you to some of the excellent resources I've discovered. Because there are so many great researchers, writers, therapists, and healers of all kinds who are making phenomenal strides in the rapidly evolving field of stress management, one of my goals in SOS is to provide referrals that will allow you to sample their good work. My hope it that these referrals will support their efforts while simultaneously getting you started on your own personal search to find the resources that are most helpful to you.

Although there are a great many excellent stress reduction tools available from which to choose, the methods I selected for *SOS: Switch Off Stress* have two traits in common:

1. Their brevity.

2. Their ease.

My objective in this book is to provide you with many tools that can provide immediate SOS relief. Your task is only this: choose one activity and DO it—*right where you are, right now.*

You certainly can spare 6 seconds to 6 minutes to stop the distress you're feeling, correct? I'm not asking you to take an hour to go to the gym or to attend a yoga class. Although both of these are both excellent stress-relievers, I know you may not be able to squeeze out that much time, especially at the moment you start feeling anxious or upset. HOWEVER, YOU CAN EASILY DO ONE OF THESE SOS TECHNIQUES at that critical point! (If not, you could be in worse shape than you realize. Read the next Background section to see why it's vital that you protect yourself from the "silent killer" of stress.)

I urge you to take any SOS activity in this book for an immediate test drive. See for yourself: I think you'll be quite surprised by how much better you feel after this "micro-vacation". In fact, I'll bet that you'll experience a terrific return for this tiny investment of your time. (SOS = great ROI.)

The 101 rapid-response activities in this book are designed to help you deal more effectively with—and recover more quickly from—small annoyances, significant aggravation, unpleasant or boring tasks, disappointments, second-hand contagion from others' stress, and real emergencies *as they occur*. I hope that, by using SOS tools in this way, you will significantly reduce any potential adverse effects of long-term, chronic, toxic stress.

Dedication: The initial copies of SOS were given as a thank you to those individuals who helped my life partner and me through our recent difficulties. We consider ourselves to be very blessed to have such good-hearted people in our lives…so allow me to make our gratitude public:

This book is dedicated to our wonderful community

of family, friends, colleagues and clients,

who formed a strong safety net of love and care

that broke our fall time and again.

And thank you for buying this book! Please use *Switch Off Stress* to augment your daily experience of happiness, health, love, and ease. And please pass on the good word about SOS relief to others. Teach some easy tools to your children so they grow up more resilient and less harmed by the pressures that surround them. Give this book as a gift to colleagues you admire and also to friends and family members you love. If you're a coach, health care provider or therapist, please share it with clients. Hand it off to a friend who's having trouble at work. If you're a teacher, use SOS to help your students excel at learning. Together, we can make your life—and that of many other people—more healthy and happy.

I invite you to join our SOS community by reading and participating in *The Balancing Act Community's Blog* (http://thecoreporation.blogspot.com) where we will share, refine, and add to the SOS tools. I would appreciate having the benefit of your knowledge, insights, and experience. And lastly, please feel free to follow me on Twitter @SharonSeivert.

Best wishes,

Sharon Seivert

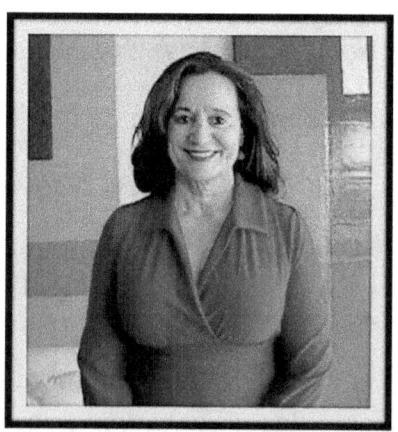

SOS: Why You Need to Stop Distress ASAP

This SOS "first-aid kit" contains a Band Aid approach to immediately relieving the pain of distress. It is not intended as cure for the root causes of your problems. It does not contain a long-term strategy for relieving chronic stress. HOWEVER, paradoxically, what this book does provide could be critical for your long-term health and success.

Almost all experts agree that distress is the number one killer in the world today and that most of our health problems have long term, physiological stress as their origin. In fact, the US Centers for Disease Control estimate that **80%** of health care dollars are spent on stress-related illnesses. Unfortunately, there is a huge gap between our collective understanding that stress contributes to illness and what we're doing collectively to address this problem. (For example, a recent survey of 5000+ American physicians indicated that only **3%** of them discussed stress management with their patients during office visits.)

My intention in writing *SOS: Switch Off Stress* is to help you cope more successfully with the everyday challenges of distress by transforming them into learning opportunities rather than have them accumulate over time into illness. (The great Austrian philosopher Rudolf Steiner called this process of slow deterioration *"calcification"*—where we become unnaturally brittle, stiff, lose our health and age more quickly.) Please use this SOS rapid-response toolkit to turn your awareness of discomfort and/or feelings of imbalance into "*moments of choice*" where you take quick, small actions that head off a host of problems (physical, mental and spiritual) instead of allowing yourself to become "calcified" by stress overload, stress accumulation, and slow recovery from distressing situations.

Switching Off Stress is important, not just for your health, but also for the health and happiness of everyone around you. Recent studies of a phenomenon called "second-hand stress" reveal that even strangers can pass on their distress to you— and visa versa (as evidenced by heart rate and cortisol level). And negative contagion effects are *four times* more likely if the people actually know each other (family, friends, co-workers).

The Morse code "SOS" was the international telegraph distress signal used during the past century as a cry for help: a ship was going down in a storm or a fort was under siege, etc. This SOS code ("...---...") has saved countless lives all over the world by getting rescuers to the emergency scene in the nick of time. I invoke this globally recognized code now, in the hopes that these *Switch Off Stress* activities will provide you with immediate, just-in-time help whenever you need it.

As pretty much everyone now knows, the same human stress response that allowed our early ancestors to survive despite incredibly hostile environments is not particularly adaptive to the subtle, chronic strains of the 21st century. In fact, over time, distress can accumulate so that it becomes hazardous to our health. The accumulation of toxic stress contributes mightily to today's leading diseases—which is one reason stress is dubbed the "silent killer". (Go to Appendix A to read more.)

To survive and thrive today, we all need a variety of tools that give us a wider range of effective options with which we can respond in our moments of distress. Sometimes a knee-jerk "fight or flight" response is absolutely appropriate—and could save your life! However, at other times it would be more effective if you deliberately pivoted to a "find and flourish" (aka a "learn and thrive") response to distress. This strategic shift could provide you not only with healthy relief in that moment; it could also create the time and space you need to discover the root causes of your problems so you can make the lasting changes necessary for you to evolve and thrive.

The Balancing Act and a Free Stress Quiz

SOS: Switch Off Stress builds on *The Balancing Act: Mastering the 5 Elements of Success in Life, Relationships and Work*, and the decade of research, development and testing that followed its publication. (See http://balance.thecorporation.com to learn about, or to purchase, *The Balancing Act* in print or as eBook.) My colleagues and I have used *The Balancing Act* (TBA) process to help our individual and group clients: a) quickly regain balance during times of acute or chronic anxiety and overwhelm; AND b) proactively change to more effective, healthier habits in order to create the lives, work, and relationships they desire.

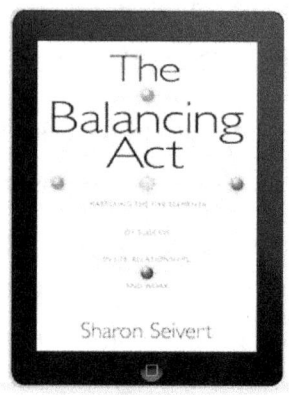

The Balancing Act (TBA) outlines an overarching meta-process, a highly effective long-term strategy for creating lasting change so you can create the life, work and relationships you desire. *SOS: Switch Off Stress* is based on TBA principles, but focuses on the immediate relief of any pressures and the removal of any obstacles that could sabotage your desired success. Practicing SOS will replenish your energy so you can learn, adapt, and stay the course—or correct it. It will also help you thoroughly enjoy each step of the journey and achieve every form of happiness. (Go to Appendix D for a synopsis and reviews of *The Balancing Act*.)

In *SOS: Switch Off Stress*, I reframe distress as a signal that you are out of balance in one or more of the 5 "Elements of Success" or Synergy. By paying attention to any weak quality, you can first strengthen it and then bring it into alignment with the other qualities. This will help you switch quickly from a state of unease and imbalance to a much more pleasant experience of greater ease and balance.

Take two-three minutes now to discover which Elements of Success are currently your most weak versus your most strong (see **Free Stress Quiz** at "thecoreporation.com" home page. You will immediately receive a short web-generated report that points to which chapters in *SOS: Switch Off Stress* are likely to have stress management activities most suited to your needs.

You can also get immediate stress relief by going directly to the chapter that is most descriptive of you (see summaries below):

Go to the following Chapter if you:

Chapter One: *Feel agitated, anxious, off-balance, uncomfortable in own skin; have low self-esteem, confidence, resilience; feel generally unhappy; take things too personally; feel unclear about life purpose, values, what's important; don't breathe deeply or sleep well; are too busy to relax or take breaks; run from one thing to the next; feel "empty" inside, not best self; have addictions can't stop (smoking, drinking, eating).*

Chapter Two: *Are bothered by mental looping, negative thinking, a hyper-active critical mind; are often doubtful, afraid, hopeless, unhappy; get stuck because over-analyze, over plan, overthink; feel uncreative, uninspired, can't generate good options; have a bad attitude, lack humor; don't enjoy things or have much fun; feel bored, unchallenged, not interested in new information/learning, don't feel as smart as used to be.*

Chapter Three: *Procrastinate too much; have a hard time figuring out priorities or making choices; feel undisciplined,*

---

dissipated, unfocused, unmotivated, overwhelmed, burned out; lack direction; reluctant to move into action or take initiative; feel micro-managed or demoralized; avoid conflict; don't feel energetic, ambitious, excited, or proud of accomplishments.

Chapter Four: *Feel emotionally "off" (overly emotional, emotionally flat, or somehow inappropriate in interactions); have key relationships that are unhealthy, unsupportive, draining, disrespectful or that keep you stuck; believe you're unappreciated, used, manipulated; are exhausted from over-giving; would rather be isolated than involved because don't feel particularly pleasant, empathetic, compassionate or caring.*

Chapter Five: *Have difficulty managing or securing sufficient money or the physical resources, space, and tools you need; are impractical, unrealistic, unorganized; have trouble following directions and keeping things orderly; can't be depended upon to complete tasks or meet deadlines; don't take good care of physical health or possessions; have dysfunctional habits that undermine what you want to create; feel unsafe, insecure.*

Chapter Six: *Are having a run of bad luck; feel less effective and balanced overall; seem to have lost good judgment, discernment, a sense of perspective; don't experience flow or ease, so things take too much time and effort; don't feel particularly grateful or happy because others are better off; lack a sense of a connection to a greater Context, Whole, Source or the infrastructures that support your work, life and relationships.*

Since the publication of *The Balancing Act*, my colleagues and I have researched, tested, and developed extensive resources and new tools that build on the TBA process. These include professional assessments, reports, books, guidebooks and full courses that provide practical, targeted help in different aspects of work, relationships and life that may be causing you distress. (These include developmental tools for: personal growth, life or career transitions, leadership, team, entrepreneurship, and organizational change.) Go to Appendix C: CORE Resources to see how TBA could help you deal with common life, relationship, and work stressors.

Make Stress Your Friend to CHANGE for Good

Is Switching off Stress as easy as turning off a light? Yes—but only if you know where that switch is! This book is designed to show you where to locate that switch inside you so you can act rapidly to stop adverse effects from excessive stress (your own or the "second-hand stress" you can catch from others).

These 101 SOS techniques will help you transform stress into a friend or teacher—not only in the emergency moment to relieve pain, but also over time, as you integrate your favorite SOS activities into your life. Here's how to use SOS to change your life for good: When you find an SOS activity you particularly enjoy, bookmark and practice it until it becomes a new habit and way of life. (After all, it is the relatively straightforward process of repeating behavior over time that forms new habits.)

With SOS, you are taking strong steps to change your life for the better by deliberately creating strong new neural pathways that turn stress triggers into "find and flourish" opportunities for discovery, evolving, and thriving. This is *neuroplasticity*, i.e., the brain's ability to change and adapt as a result of experience. (Although previously it was believed that our brains had pretty much formed before adulthood, we now know they continue to create new neural pathways and alter existing ones. So there are no excuses: you can always adapt to new experiences, learn new information, and create new memories.)

I hope you'll use SOS to help your brain form healthier new patterns, i.e., replace less-effective stress responses with more functional SOS techniques. I recommend that you change just one habit at a time; that way it can settle in so you can gage its effects. Then, **after you've incorporated that first SOS activity into your life, choose a next new healthy habit to adopt. These small changes are very powerful; indeed, tiny new habits can transform your life in wonderful ways in very little time.**

From 6 seconds to 6 minutes to no time at all. In fact, I have some great news: many of these SOS tools will take you NO time at all once you've learned them. (Really.) You can easily do many SOS techniques while you're doing other things (walking, working, waiting, commuting, listening, doing housework, etc.) In fact, I find that these stress management actions can reduce my resistance, and in this way make difficult duties or boring tasks easier for me. Also, you can replace any neutral or bad habit you currently have (that likely wastes plenty of valuable time) with one of SOS's much healthier and more efficient new habits.

Changing for good. The process of creating new habits is reflected in the steps of *The Balancing Act*'s powerful CHANGE model. These steps—which significantly increase your odds of making sustainable change—are encoded in the spiral image below (each step reflects one of the chapters in this book):

Step 1. Reset (Core)

Step 2. Reframe (Vision)

Step 3. Reprioritize (Mission)

Step 4. Relate (Interactions)

Step 5. Repeat (Structure)

Step 6. Reform (Synergy)

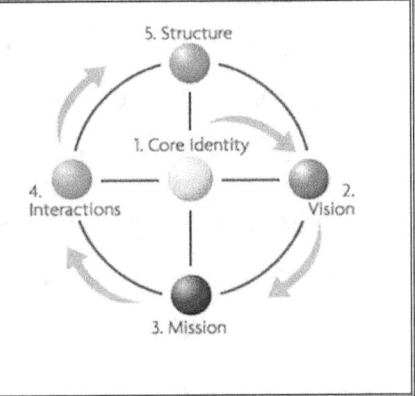

See Appendix A: Make Stress Your Friend to Change for Good.

Get the Most from *Switch Off Stress*

If you read About the Author in Appendix B, you will learn that I've written a fair number of books. This one, by far, has been THE most fun—and I hope you enjoy using it as much as I enjoyed having to test and retest these stress reduction tools. Poor me: laughing, stretching, breathing, and doing happiness techniques. What's not to love?

I hope you'll agree. I consider these SOS activities to be "micro-vacations"—which could provide you with more positive impact than regular vacations. In fact, the benefits from a standard (American) two-week vacation tend to dissipate within a few days after getting back to work. In contrast, I find that I can take several refreshing SOS breaks every day—which add up to a whole lot more of my life feeling as if I am on vacation.

How to use this book: 1) Take the free Stress Quiz at thecoreporation.com to discover which element needs the most help; 2) choose an SOS technique that fits within the time you have available; 3) randomly pick an activity to try; or, 4) work systematically through the whole book.

Go to Section I: To find "how to" instructions for each SOS rapid-response tool; for help with a particular Element of Success, go to that chapter in Section I.

Go to Section II: To learn more about an SOS activity, you can see more details here about that technique (why it works, what it can do for you, and where you can find more resources).

Go to Section III: For more information about SOS's author, background, research and resources.

Go to Online Resources: For direct links to SOS instructions.

Special note: If you are currently injured or ill, or if you are a person with a disability, please feel free to adapt instructions throughout SOS so it serves you better.

Please use this book only for the purposes intended (disclaimer). This book is designed to educate and entertain by providing information about distress and instructions about ways to relieve it. It is sold with the understanding that the publisher and author are NOT engaged in rendering medical, coaching, therapeutic, or other professional services. The author and CORE Press shall have neither liability nor responsibility to any person or entity with respect to any loss or damage caused or alleged to be caused directly or indirectly by information contained in this book.

The information provided throughout this book is NOT offered as medical advice. It is vital that you do not use this book as a substitute for, or as an excuse to delay seeking, medical or mental health treatment.

Go immediately to the appropriate health care provider if you are experiencing physical, mental or emotional symptoms of distress. I also suggest that you have regular medical and mental health check-ins; this is a powerful preventative strategy to avoid harm from the silent killer of stress.

Every effort has been made to make this book as complete and accurate as possible. However, if you find errors (typos, content, defunct links), please send corrections to "sseivert" @ "thecoreporation.com" for the next edition of *SOS: Switch Off Stress*. Thank you!

SECTION I:

FIRST AID INSTRUCTIONS

FOR

101 SOS TECHNIQUES

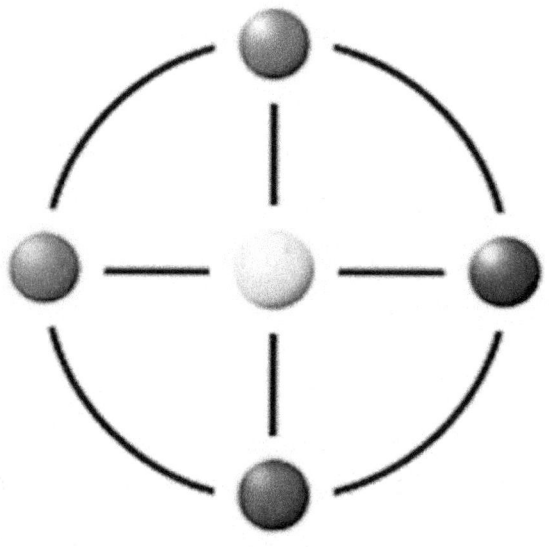

Chapter One:

Strengthen Your Core

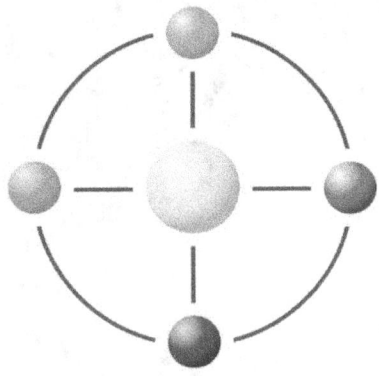

The techniques in this first chapter will help you reduce stress so you: feel more centered and calm; increase your self-esteem; become more creative and productive; feel very comfortable in your own skin; don't take things so personally; become clearer about values and what matters most to you; be certain you are acting ethically and staying true to yourself.

The Core is first Element of Success. In *The Balancing Act,* your Core corresponds to the Center of the wheel (as in the image above), the classical element of Essence, and your Soul. You can think of Core as being your own internal sun, around which all the other moving parts of your life rotate. It is your personal self-referencing, gravitational center-point; as such, it keeps you feeling balanced and happy rather than off-balance and out of sorts. This first element is subtle, invisible, but very real and powerful; it is the "essential" force that holds everything else together in your life, relationships, and work.

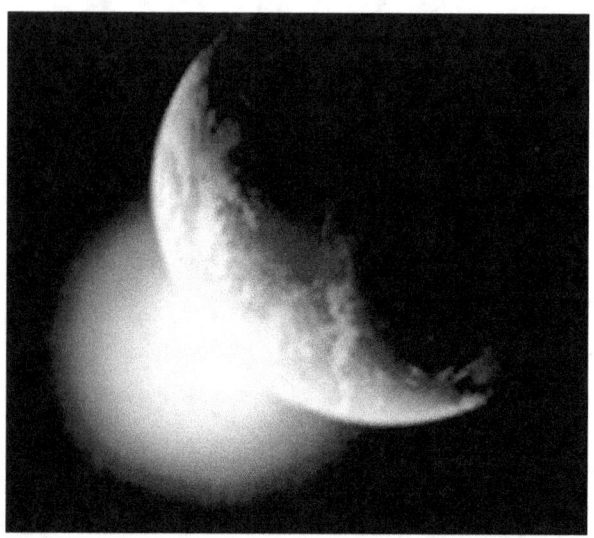

The Core element is "who you are" when you're feeling at your best. It includes your non-negotiable principles and ethics, your truest self (core identity and values—both personally and professionally), your intuitive intelligence, and the native gifts that make you special. Ancient Greek philosophers described your Core as an *in-dwelling spirit*—and compared it to a deeply buried golden figurine, a priceless, internal treasure. When you uncover this Core of yourself, they said, you will experience *eudaemonic* (purpose-driven) happiness and be able to thrive.

A strong Core optimizes creativity and productivity in work and life. In fact, the fast SOS activities noted in this Core chapter will allow you to pause at critical moments so you can renew your energy and increase your odds of staying at the top of your game. When you are centered, you feel at home in your own skin, even during difficult times. A strong Core helps you cope better by making you unflappable, calm, and happy in a *self-referenced* way (independent of external circumstances). It also helps you make sustainable changes by insisting you start from the inside and then move out. This element functions much like a steady, experienced driver who knows where you want to go and also the best possible route to get you there.

All these reasons make this first element a great place to begin if you want to *Switch Off Stress*. The Core launches the upward Spiral of Synergy by forcing you to STOP, i.e., pause, center, breathe, and release distress before you even think about moving forward. This first step also ensures that the TBA Change process starts positively, with short, refreshing "times-out" that can RESET your life.

Dealing with potentially toxic stress in this way makes you a real-life hero: i.e., someone who is willing to venture into uncharted internal territory to discover the golden treasure that is buried there. *For more information about the Core Element of Success, read pages 35-48 in The Balancing Act.* (To read more about TBA, go to http://balance.thecoreporation.com.)

SOS Techniques that Strengthen Your Core:

1. Experience the Calming Core Element (p 32)
2. Stealth Breath (p 33)
3. Walking Breath (p 34)
4. Emergency Breath (p 36)

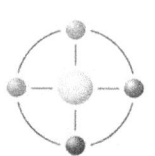

#1: Experience the Calming Core Element

(4-6 minutes)

<u>How to do SOS #1:</u> Go to thecoreporation.com home page (or the sos_links page) and click on the Core meditation audio. Then sit back, listen to my voice, and let me do all the work.

Go to Section II to learn more (p 179).

#2: Stealth Breath

(2-4 minutes)

How to do SOS #2: A relatively easy way to center and experience the profoundly calming quality of your internal Core is by using a variety of simple breathing techniques. This first one is a basic breath count that I call the *stealth breath* (because nobody has to know you're doing it).

The reason to do a count with your breathing is so you notice how shallowly you are breathing in response to any perceived threat. After you become aware of your breath, you can use any of the below counting techniques to slow it down and instantaneously countermand any distress signals you may unwittingly be sending your brain and body. The counting is a way to keep you from "cheating" when you're first learning how to deliberately deepen and elongate your breathing.

There are many versions of this technique, but I recommend that you start very simply: just stop whatever you're doing and sit quietly while breathing deeply in and slowly out.

Option One:

Count slowly to yourself…

"Breathe in – 2 – 3 - 4"; "Breathe Out - 2- 3- 4." (Repeat.)

Option Two:

Add pauses between inhalation and exhalation.

Option Three:

Exhale longer than you inhale.

"Breathe In – 2 – 3; Breathe Out – 2 – 3 – 4 – 5." (Repeat).

You can breathe in and out through your nose, OR you can breathe in through your nose and out through your mouth. Experiment with these different options and choose whatever is most comfortable for you. As thoughts come into your mind, just notice them, say "Thanks for bringing that to my attention", and then return to the count and your breath. When your mind is finally quiet, you can let go of the count and simply enjoy the internal silence and mental peace.

One of the beauties of this silent practice is that nobody has to know you're doing it—hence the *stealth* label. For example, you can use it to increase alertness and remain calm while listening more attentively during boring meetings or to calm yourself while you're on an unsettling phone call. In fact, this simple, highly portable technique is a good one to use as your default "go-to" stress manager. *Go to Section II to learn more (p 179).*

#3: Walking Breath

(5- 6 minutes)

<u>How to do SOS #3:</u> This is a variation of the "Stealth" Breath count (SOS #2). However, in this technique, you will use your steps to keep time with the breath count. When you notice that you are agitated, all you have to do is get up from your desk

and start your stealth count walk-about. Just breathe in and out deeply and steadily while silently counting in pace with your walking steps, for example:

"Breathe In" (first step) – "2" (next step) – "3" (third step)…

"Breathe Out (next steps) – "2" – "3" – "4" – "5".

(Repeat counting in time with steps. Note: depending on how fast you walk, you may take two steps per breath count.)

As thoughts come into your mind, just notice them, release them, and return your attention to your breath count and steps. Your mind needs to focus on walking and avoiding bumping into things while simultaneously counting your breath in and out. This technique will keep you sufficiently busy so you'll find it difficult to even recall distressing thoughts.

After 5-6 minutes, when you mind is quiet, you can let go of the count and simply enjoy the internal silence, mental peace, fresh air and scenery as you walk. Once you get the hang of this activity, you can easily turn it into a "no-time-at-all" SOS technique because you have to walk to places anyway. Transform your walking into a "don't hurry-don't worry" steady, sane pace by which you glide gracefully and happily to your destination. *Go to Section II to learn more (p 181).*

#4: Emergency Breath

(10-20 seconds)

<u>*How to do SOS #4:*</u> There are many ways to do emergency breathing to help out in extreme stress situations. This is a highly effective, three-step power-breathing process. Note: At first, do this technique only a) in a place where you will not disturb others, and b) while sitting or lying down, as it could make you light-headed.

Step 1 (optional): The Pretzel. Put your arms straight out in front of you. Cross your wrists with palms facing. Then interlace your fingers and tuck your hands back under your wrists, so they point toward your body. Rest interlaced hands gently on your chest. This pretzel pose is odd, but it engages your whole brain to provide extra benefits from this technique. Take a few slow breaths to settle down and center before moving on.

Step 2: Power Breathing. Do "power-breathing" for 10 seconds. This means taking fast, deep and full belly-breaths, so the whole trunk of your body moves. The breathing is from your mouth and is rather noisy. (Slow down your breathing if you feel light-headed or start to hyperventilate.)

Step 3: Refocus. While doing the emergency breathing, take your mind off the stressor and focus it instead on something positive—for example, imagine a good outcome to this situation or think about someone you love.

Optional: To realize the strong impact of this technique, rate the stress you're feeling from 1-10, both before and after doing it.

You can use this "ER" Breath either as: a) an effective rapid-response technique to stop extreme stress, or b) a daily preventive, "time-out" technique to clear your body and mind from any stress residue. In fact, doing the ER breath 3x/day can bring all kinds of health benefits. And since it only takes 10-20 seconds per round, it's a small time investment for a great return. Try it out a few times and you'll quickly see how much it can help you. *Go to Section II to learn more (p 182).*

#5: Soothing Sounds

(5-6 minutes—or as long as you wish)

How to do SOS #5: Just find a soothing video or audio you like, sit back, listen, and melt into a pool of peace and contentment. Set your alarm for the amount of time you have available for this "soothing sounds" relaxing micro-vacation. My clients and I have had great success using such aids to ease us into sleep or meditation.

I have noted direct links to a wide range of soothing music at "thecoreporation.com/sos_links". You can also put key words into YouTube, sign up for relaxation and meditation channels, go to online radio stations such as AccuRadio (see Textures), ITunes, and many other web resources. Once you find artists and types of soothing sounds you particularly enjoy, you can buy, bookmark, or/or download them onto your computer, mobile device or home sound system for instant SOS relief whenever you need it.

And you may find that you'd like to use soothing sounds, not just as a time-out, but also as background music that is interwoven into the natural fabric of your day. I regularly use calm, non-verbal music while I'm working—which into a "no time at all" SOS technique that significantly improves my creativity and increases my productivity.

Here are some suggested key words to launch your search: *Sleep, Relaxation, Meditation, Classical music for meditation, Study music, Native American Music, Gentle Rain, Ocean, Zen Garden. Go to Section II to learn more (p 183).*

#6: Small Universe

(5-6 minutes)

How to do SOS #6: This is an abbreviated version of a very powerful Qigong meditation, as taught by Dr. Chunyi Lin (see *Learn More* for a referral to Dr. Lin' remarkable work). Even though this version is simplified, it will still go a long way to reducing your stress and increasing your energy.

Begin by touching the tip of your tongue to the roof of your mouth as you smile slightly, take a deep breath in, and say to yourself: "I am in the universe. The universe is in my body. The universe and I combine together." Then imagine deeply breathing in energy to each of these spots as you take a full tour around your body (your own "small universe").

You begin this breathing process by bringing your attention to the first spot, which is deep behind your navel (the "lower dantian"); this is where we start and end each full round. Imagine that you are deeply breathing in the purest energy to this point. Then, as you slowly breathe out, imagine pushing that energy to the next spot, your bladder area.

Breathe in deeply to your bladder area and imagine breathing out that energy to the next spot, which is at the bottom of your torso between your legs. And so this process continues as you breathe deeply in and slowly out of each below-listed spot:

Breathe in to the bottom of torso, and then out to the tailbone.
Breathe in to the tailbone, and then out to the small of the back.
(…Breathe IN…Breathe OUT)
…small of back…kidney area.
…kidney area…neck.
…neck…base of skull.
…base of skull…top of head.
…top of head…3rd eye (forehead).
…3rd eye…throat.
…throat…heart.
…heart…naval.
(Now you've completed one full round.)

Repeat the Small Universe process as often as you wish. I find it very invigorating. *Go to Section II to learn more (p 184).*

#7: Countdown

(2 minutes)

How to do SOS #7: Find a comfortable position, close your eyes, take a deep breath through your nose and, as you exhale through your mouth, mentally repeat and visualize the numbers as noted in the countdown options below.

Option One:

Take a deep breath in. Then as you slowly exhale, mentally repeat and visualize the number "3" three times:

"3 --- 3 ---3" (pause)

Take another deep breath in, and then as you slowly exhale, mentally repeat and visualize the number "2" three times:

"2 --- 2 ---2" (pause)

Take another deep breath in and as you slowly exhale, mentally repeat and visualize the number "1" three times:

"1 --- 1 ---1" (pause)

Option Two:

As you silently say and see the number "3", you can increase your focus by imagining that you are changing the internal volume from medium to soft to very soft; you could also change the size of the number you see, from large to medium to small.

Option Three:

I have also used this countdown technique by starting at the number "10" or "5" and counting down slowly to "1".

Option Four:

Another highly effective variation on the countdown is to mentally see yourself stepping into an elevator at the 10th floor, and then slowly, smoothly descending as you visualize the numbers on the elevator panel lighting up to mark each floor. While imagining your descent, you can instruct yourself to become more relaxed with each lower floor. When you arrive completely relaxed at the ground floor, the doors will open and you can move forward with your day, feeling great.

BTW: Do not underestimate the value of this technique because it's so simple. Just try it out for yourself.

Go to Section II to learn more (p 185).

#8: Access Your GPS

(4-6 minutes)

<u>How to do SOS #8:</u> You have your own, already-installed "GPS" that is a reliable guide to dealing with stress—all you have to do is to access it. This internal GPS system is your Core's deep intuitive intelligence—which is exponentially more effective than the rationale cognitive processes you have probably been relying on for problem solving.

Start this technique by getting quiet for a few minutes. In our noise-filled era, that is not a state with which you're likely to be comfortable at first. However, your internal GPS is constantly processing information and trying to send you directions that, unfortunately, are usually drowned out in day-to-day activity. Now your new friend, Stress, is urging you to turn off your busy Mind for a few moments so you can listen to these signals.

There are many techniques for accessing your internal GPS, several of which are noted in this Core SOS chapter. After one or two minutes of a Core breath technique, your Mind will become more calm and receptive as it takes a short break from analyzing and worrying about the issue you're trying to resolve.

Then, ask yourself the question for which you want GPS guidance. Use your breath to remain centered. Wait for an impulse to come from your "gut" (this is where people often feel intuition in their bodies). Sometimes an answer will pop into your quieted mind as a nonverbal impulse—much like a stone creates ripples in a still pond. At other times you may hear a deep internal voice answering "yes" or "no" to your question. And sometimes a completely unexpected idea pops up that you wouldn't have thought of otherwise. Have paper and a pen handy to write down whatever comes, even if it is a surprise.

After you access your intuition to manage distress a few times, it will become clearer which feedback is intuitive intelligence and which comes from your rationale mind. What you're doing with this SOS activity is connecting your Core to a limitless source of information that provides a wider range of options. This process will make certain you don't inadvertently select out data that could be helpful or miss an intuitive breakthrough.

Don't be discouraged if this GPS technique doesn't work the first time or two you try it. (Think of it as reestablishing communication with an old friend you've ignored for many years. It's well worth reaching out until the two of you are both talking again.) Other ways to access your Intuition are noted elsewhere in this SOS First Aid Kit. A few I recommend are:

- Talk to Your Smartest Self (SOS #15)

- Green—Yellow—Red Light (SOS #63)

- Take a Nature Break (SOS #82)

Go to Section II to learn more (p 186).

#9: Sing those Blues Away

(3-4 minutes)

How to do SOS #9: You can sing in the shower, while commuting in your car, join a choir, and whistle while you work, or grab the mike at karaoke night. No matter how or where you do it, just do it! Singing forces you to breathe—AND it makes breathing so much more fun. It is one of the all-time greatest stress relievers. And it's fast: singing along to many popular songs takes only three minutes or so. There's hardly any faster way to switch from stress to unabashed joy.

Personally, I love to belt out a blues song, sing my own songs, or choose an upbeat pop melody or a classic show tune to sing-along (now you know all my secrets). Go to AccuRadio, YouTube, or other online radio stations to explore different channels and find the best music for chasing away your blues. And if you're stuck in a place where you could lose your job or freedom if you sang at the top of your lungs, you may be able to listen with a headset so you don't disturb anyone.

To jump-start this activity, you can sing or dance along with these great happiness anthems: "Don't Worry, Be Happy" by Bobby McFeein (feature=player_ detailpage&v=d-diB65scQU) and "Happy" (v=y6Sxv-sUYtM) by Pharrell Williams. *Go to Section II for lyrics and to learn more (p 187).*

#10: Beam Me Up

(2-3 minutes)

<u>How to do SOS #10:</u> When you're feeling overwhelmed or depleted, this is a great de-stressing and reenergizing technique. You can do it lying down, sitting at your desk, in a boring meeting, or while walking outdoors. Start by focusing on your breath until you're internally quiet. Then imagine connecting with a column of light (any color you prefer) that is coming from hundreds of feet above you, directly into the top of your head. With each breath, imagine that you are allowing the light to continue through your body, starting at the top of your skull and then slowly moving down your face, spine, trunk,

core, arms and legs, filling up every cell of your body with renewed energy. (If you wish, you can image that you're exhaling any toxins you feel inside; this makes certain the light you're breathing in seeps into every tiny corner of you.)

This should be a pleasant, gentle exercise that combines your breath with deliberate positive imagining; please enjoy it to the fullest. It's fantastic to do when you are outdoors, so you can enjoy the sunshine that much more. You can stop this exercise when you're "all filled up" with light. Better now? (I thought so.) *Go to Section II to learn more (p 189).*

#11: Lightning Strikes

(3-4 minutes)

How to do SOS #11: If you need a very strong energy boost, you can do a variation of Beam Me Up (SOS #10). Here you would continue past the point of feeling all filled up with light. That is, you will allow the beam of light you've imagined to continue through you until it sinks deeply into the ground.

And, if you're feeling adventurous, you can mentally propel that light beam all the way to the center of the earth—and then have it bounce back to you (almost as if from a trampoline). This way you will feel the deep, rich energy of the earth combine with the energy from the heavens, meeting halfway, powerfully, in your heart center. (This activity reflects how lighting actually occurs:

i.e., an equal force from above and below connect in the middle to create the explosion of a lightning strike.)

Lastly, imagine that the combined energies from above and below fill you with pulsing light and expand outward to form a circle of light all around you. By now you should feel completely regenerated, with your stress totally blasted away.

Optional: If you want to continue even further, you can imagine this powerful light expanding to fill the room you're in and your whole home. And then you can expand it so it moves through your town, state, country, the world, and out into the universe. After these 2 or 3 additional expansive minutes, you will feel even more happy, connected, and at peace. *Go to Section II to learn more (p 189).*

#12: Breathe a Smile In — Breathe Toxins Out

(10-20 seconds)

How to do SOS #12: This technique is so easy that you could overlook its power and skip it. That would be a mistake, especially since it takes mere seconds to do.

As you breathe in through your nose, smile slightly. Direct each smiling inhalation to soften and soothe any places in your body where you have tension, pain, discomfort or tiredness. Then, with each long exhalation through your mouth, imagine relaxing your whole body as you breathe out all tiredness, tension, specific pain, or discouraging and negative thoughts.

46

Repeat as often as you wish: Smile softly while breathing in; relax your whole body while breathing out toxins and pain.

Happily, this is another stealth SOS technique that can be done anywhere, anytime, and anyplace to help you feel noticeably better in seconds. *Go to Section II to learn more (p 190).*

#13: Call a Time Out

(90 seconds)

How to do SOS #13: When you were acting out as a child, did your parents demand that you take a "time out"? Mine did. And, although I hated being called out on my bad behavior, invariably I felt much better after they gave me this unrequested break. (And most certainly, so did everyone else.) This activity requires only that your inner parents notice when you're spinning out of control. It requires just a few seconds to first recognize the danger signals that you're out-of-balance, and then only a minute more to counter balance by temporarily walking away (physically or mentally) from the situation.

In addition to good parenting, the other area time-outs are relied upon is sports. For example, taking a time out is a wise strategy when the game is on the line and the team needs to huddle to adjust its strategy—or, when there's only a few seconds with one free throw left to win the game, and the star player needs a vital moment to catch her breath.

Become your own caring parent or coach. Observe yourself, notice when stress is adversely affecting you, then enforce your own times-out. For example, all you may need to do for a great time-out is to unplug yourself from all your electronic devices for a few moments. (A great idea!) Or you can simply close your eyes and breathe for a bit. Or, you can get up from your desk and walk around the block for a pleasant way to get unstuck, refresh and restart. Push back on the stress of deadlines by carving out regular break times so you work and think more effectively. It's actually good for business! Indeed, research proves that taking a time-out actually *increases* productivity. (See cnn.com/ 2014/05/16/opinion/schulte-daydreaming-productivity/). It is also vital to creativity because "Ah-ha" breakthrough insights occur when we allow ourselves to "oscillate" between times of focused attention and relaxation.

All the Core SOS activities are particularly useful in helping you counter-balance moments of high pressure with effective relaxation. These will quickly rebalance you so you can return to work renewed. I also recommend treating your senses during time-out breaks (see SOS #81).

Whatever you do, use your "times-out" to (metaphorically) go to the corner, play out doors, stop picking on others, and/or get yourself out of everyone's hair. The kinds of time-out I'm recommending are *rewards,* not punishments. They create deliberate pivot points that allow you to shift from stress to success when you most need to do so. These "smart-breaks" acknowledge the pressure you're under and provide immediate benefits by having you take good care of yourself. Decide how to make them enjoyable treats. Have some fun. Do different things. Mix it up. *Go to Section II to learn more (p 190).*

#14: No More Waiting to Exhale

(<6 seconds)

How to do SOS #14: Whenever you realize that you're holding your breath because you're stressed–don't wait! Simply exhale as much air as you possibly can from your lungs. Breathe out through your mouth until your lungs are like completely deflated balloons with no air at all remaining in them.

You can also do a proactive exhalation by modifying the SOS Core breath count techniques so that you *start* your breath count with the exhalation and make the exhalation longer than the inhalation. (In yogic practice it's said that if you take care of the exhalation, the inhalation will take care of itself.) Another way to do this is with silent verbal signals, such as: "Breathe out looooooooooong. Pause. Breathe in deep. Pause."

By exhaling longer than inhaling, you remove the carbon dioxide and toxins in your system that can build up and reduce lung capacity over time. It's a bit like opening up all the windows in your house so you establish a healthy, ongoing circulation that continually draws in clean, fresh air and pushes stale air out. *Go to Section II to learn more (p 192).*

#15: Talk to your Smartest Self

(5-6 minutes)

How to do SOS #15: Self-dialogue is an excellent way to reduce stress. With this SOS technique you let go of trying to figure things out all by yourself, and instead direct your Core to find an answer to a stressful or resistant problem by accessing your "in-tuition", i.e., by talking to the smartest part of yourself.

Keep an attractive journal and a nice pen close at hand so you can record the answers that come from this self-dialogue. Write a question at top of the page. By doing so, you set the stage to have an internal dialogue with your instinctive intelligence.

Sit quietly. Breathe easily in and out. Empty your mind of any thoughts as they pop up. Keep your pen lightly in your hand, resting its point gently at the top of the page. After a minute or two, you are likely to get an impulse to start writing, perhaps in an almost stream-of-consciousness way. If nothing comes to you after a couple minutes, just start writing and see where it leads you. Follow this internal conversation wherever it goes.

You know you're on the right track when: a) the answers are surprising but have a good gut feel to them; b) advice seems to be from your best nature—kind, gentle, respectful, responsible; and c) the answers come as advice that is conversationally addressed to "you". *Go to Section II to learn more (p 193).*

#16: Make a Space around the Pain

(2-3 minutes)

How to do SOS #16: When you're feeling mental, emotional or physical pain, sometimes you can "make a space" around that pain to lessen its negative impact.

Option One:

Let's say you have a tight knot in your shoulders. Direct your Mind to visualize that tense spot, and then imagine breathing directly into and out of it. Ease the tension with each inhalation and exhalation. You could also see yourself shining a light on that spot so you can create a ring of light and space around it. Then imagine breathing out that tension, so that spot inside becomes more and more light.

The analogy is that, much like shining a bright torch in a cave, you are bringing your consciousness into that dark space—and by so doing, chasing away many of the shadows.

Repeat this process as often as it takes to get some relief. (You can apply this technique to physical, mental or emotional pain.)

Option Two:

An alternate approach is: rather than fighting or resisting this discomfort, make a deliberate decision to simply accept it as "what is" right now. This doesn't mean that you have to like this pain, or that you're giving up hope, or that you don't intend to get to the root of this problem and change it. What this optional pain-relief strategy *does* mean is that you are going to take a break from railing against the current reality. The paradox is: if you do decide to accept "what is" in this one particular moment, it is likely that the pain will not bother you quite as much as it did the moment before. *Go to Section II to learn more (p 193).*

#17: Sounds and Silence

(4 minutes)

How to do SOS #17: Sit in a spot where you will not be disturbed for a few moments. You could close the door to your office, silence your phone, or sit on a bench in a park.

1st Minute: Use a Core breathing technique to become quiet.

2nd Minute: Scan the many sounds that you hear around you. Choose one and focus on it. Bring that sound fully into your awareness. Notice that whatever you pay attention to shifts to the "foreground", while everything else seems to subside. Nothing has changed except your deliberate observation. Notice how much more sharply, clearly, and loudly you hear this one particular sound on which you are now focused.

3rd Minute: Return your attention to your breath and then turn your listening focus to a different sound, one that was previously a background noise. Focus on it until it comes to the foreground and all other noises recede.

4th Minute: After switching back and forth a few times, see if you can "hear" the silence that is the background space that surrounds you. That silence is ephemeral but always present, a bit like the slight pause between your breaths.

This all-encompassing background silence may give you a profoundly peaceful sensation that is similar to the experience of gazing at the velvet darkness that encases millions of stars in the night sky. *Go to Section II to learn more (p 194).*

Chapter Two:

Soothe Your Mind

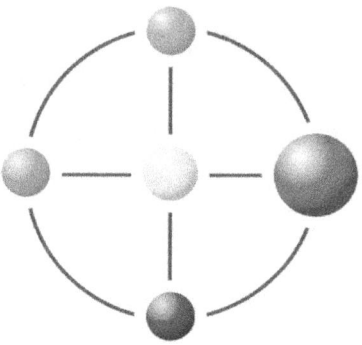

The techniques in this chapter will reduce stress by helping you gain more control over your mind. Then you'll feel more inspired and innovative; be better humored, positive and happier; generate more hopes than fears about your future; learn from experience so you can adapt and thrive; plan more effectively; access your intelligence and become more knowledgeable in areas that are important to you.

Vision is the second Element of Success. In *The Balancing Act,* Vision corresponds to the Mind of a human being, the inspiring, uplifting element of Air, and the direction of East (where the sun rises, bringing each brand new day).

Vision includes your personal beliefs and worldview, cognitive intelligence/IQ, hopes and fears, inventiveness and level of optimism, hope and happiness. It also is reflected in a positive attitude and a capacity or willingness to learn and adapt. Vision also shows up in your knowledge and professional expertise.

This element helps you imagine and then create the ideal scenarios for every aspect of your work, life and relationships. Indeed, when this Element is functioning well, you may feel as if the sky is the limit.

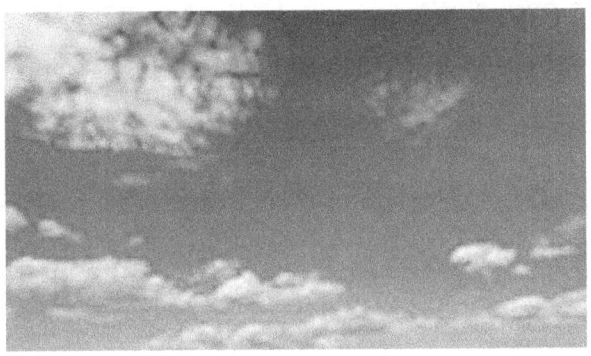

Unfortunately, Vision gets clouded when you're feeling anxious—it's hard to think clearly. You start imagining the worst possible outcomes; you may suddenly feel afraid, doubtful, stuck, or have trouble concentrating and be easily distracted.

The second Element of Success addresses fears and prevents the build up of potentially toxic stress by showing you which obstacles are illusory (so you can stop obsessing) versus which are real (so you can figure out how to deal with them head-on). All the SOS activities in this chapter will help you "stop and think". This second step in the upward Spiral of Synergy prevents or relieves distress by making certain your Mind is always directed by your Core, i.e., your best, most intelligent, centered, calm self.

In the TBA Change process, Vision is the second step that helps you "Reframe" your thinking. It deliberately shifts your mind's focus so you perceive things differently, consciously choose more functional beliefs, and move from your fears toward your hopes. That way you can focus on what you DO want to happen rather than what you dread. *For more about Vision, read pages 68-84 in The Balancing Act.* (To learn more about TBA, see http://balance.thecoreporation.com.)

SOS Techniques that Soothe Your Mind:

18. Experience the Inspiring Vision Element (p 57)
19. STOP IT! (p 57)
20. Take a Laughter Break (p 58)
21. Slow down your Brain Waves (p 60)
22. The Tetris Effect (p 61)
23. Get Inspired (p 63)
24. Time Travel (Anticipation & Memories) (p 64)
25. Mirror of the Mind (p 66)
26. C'mon, Get Happy! (p 67)
27. How Much Will this Matter...? (p 68)
28. How Did You Contribute to This? (p 69)
29. Mental Shielding (p 70)
30. Subliminal Stress Relief (p 72)
31. Reframe Stress as a Friend and Teacher (p 72)
32. Give Your Eyes a Break (p 74)
33. Participant/Observer Dual Lens (p 75)
34. Observe, Ask, Learn, Adapt (p 76)

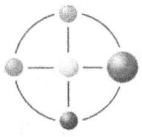

#18: Experience the Inspiring Vision Element

(6 minutes)

How to do SOS #18: Go to thecoreporation.com home page (or the sos_links page) and click on the Vision meditation audio. Then sit back, listen to my voice, and let me do all the work. *Go to Section II to learn more (p 195).*

#19: STOP IT!

(<6 second to 6-minute versions)

How to do SOS #19: There are several versions of this SOS technique from which you can choose:

<6-second version: When your mind is looping with catastrophic or unproductive thoughts, command yourself to "Stop It!" It takes only a few seconds to reverse your stress by commanding your mind to STOP, then breathing deeply in and out a few times. Listen to the silence and feel the peace that remains after you've ordered these negative thoughts to stop. (Ahhhh…yes…now that feels much better, doesn't it?)

10-second version: When you catch yourself having a negative thought, you can say (out loud if possible): "Well, that was unpleasant and unnecessary". (A command to "cut it out".)

60-second version: Another way to "Stop it" is to imagine a light switch that represents the stress you're feeling. See it as clearly as you possibly can: color, shape, size. Then take a deep breath, and in your mind's eye, walk over to it and turn it off. Voila—you've just Switched Off Stress!

2-4 minute version: In the space between sleeping and waking, order yourself to stop worrying and instead direct your mind to remember the good things that happened that day and/or how good you feel in this soft in-between moment.

6-minute version: Watch this famous Bob Newhart video (v=MDpyS2HN5SA). Here Newhart plays a therapist with a unique—and hilarious—approach. My Dutch colleague, Jan Stoop, sent this video to me years ago with the comment that this was the most effective coaching advice he had ever heard. It certainly is the funniest. I hope you enjoy it too.

Since my first viewing of this video, I have shared it with many clients, much to their delight. "Stop It!" has even become a code phrase that my colleagues, clients and I use to recall this powerful, yet often ignored, stress-remedy when we most need it. *Go to Section II to learn more (p 196).*

#20: Take a Laughter Break

(2-4 minutes)

<u>How to do SOS #20:</u> This is one of the most simple, and certainly the most entertaining stress-stoppers in this whole

book. Laughter has many health benefits that mimic a good workout. Indulge yourself in a soft chuckle or a knee-slapping Laugh out Loud. Do you have any particularly good-natured entertaining colleagues, friends or family members? If so, take some time out with them. For example, I consider my sister Irene to be one of the funniest people I know. I know that if I call her, she will soon lift my spirits and get me laughing.

Another laughter-break option is to watch a funny YouTube video or find websites that feature your favorite comedians and sitcoms. Some of my favorite laugh sites are *The Daily Show*; SNL programs old and new (particular during election years); *Whose Line is it Anyway?*; CNN Distraction; funny animal or baby videos; and late-night comedians' commentaries on news events. Your next hearty laugh is only a click or two away.

For longer laughter breaks, you can watch classic comedy movies and TV shows that suit your tastes. Bookmark, tape or purchase whatever most tickles your unique funny bone so you can watch them anytime you need a good laugh.

Another way to take a laughter break is to laugh out loud with someone else. Laughter is contagious: this is why laughter tracks are used in sitcoms and why anyone in the vicinity of a laughing person is likely to join in, making it more and more difficult for anyone involved to stop. (See Laughter Yoga, SOS #60, and Learn More for laughter links.) *Go to Section II to learn more (p 197).*

#21: Slow Down Your Brain Waves

(1-2 minutes)

How to do SOS #21: When you're feeling upset, anxious, angry, or overwhelmed, stop for just a moment and observe your thoughts. Notice what emotions are tied to these stressful thoughts. An emotion is a personal "like" or "dislike" that you attach to a thought. The stronger your personal like or dislike is, the stronger your emotion. What's more, the stronger your emotion, the higher the frequency of the brain wave that is attached to that disruptive thought…and the more stressful that thought is to your personal balancing act. The good news is that you can reverse this unhealthy chain reaction by deliberately slowing down your brain waves. Here's how:

Use any of the Core techniques to interrupt the highly charged thought and keep it from looping. If you're in a panic, use the emergency breath (SOS #4) to get your thoughts under control. And, if prior trauma is contributing to this emotionally-charged thinking, I urge you to try SOS #53 or SOS #54 to separate the emotion from the thought so you can feel calm right now, plus reduce the odds of re-triggering this negative chain reaction.

The ideal brainwave frequency when you are relaxed or meditating is **10** brain cycles per second (alpha). When you're awake, the ideal brainwave frequency (beta) is approximately **20** cycles per second. However, the more emotional your thoughts become, the higher your brain wave frequency. For example, if you're angry or afraid, your brain wave frequency could rise to **30** or above. That's when you "see red" and are more likely to do something you'll regret. (See Red Flag, SOS #74.) Then you'll find it harder to remedy that stress because you're thinking less and less clearly as your brain wave frequency rises. *Go to Section II to learn more (p 198).*

#22: The Tetris Effect

(2-4 minutes)

How to do SOS #22: The *"Tetris Effect"* was first coined when dedicated players of the video game Tetris would stop after hours of playing, but then perceive the patterns of this game superimposed onto the real world. The name was later used for any habit-forming mental activity that develops patterns that can overshadow people's thoughts, images or dreams.

In most modern cultures, we are trained to be hyper-vigilant for danger and errors, i.e., we scan for negative patterns as a way to protect ourselves. Unfortunately, the more we scan for mistakes, typos, problems, muggers, and potential catastrophes—the more we train our brains to focus on them. This habit can make the Tetris Effect a highly stressful, selectively negative lens. Over time, we create and reinforce neural pathways and develop perceptual patterns where we, sadly, no longer notice all the good that's going on all around us. The unintended consequence is that we do not observe and therefore cannot leverage the best of what's available to us. In a way, we become blind to—and cut off from—the positive.

There is a relevant quote from the Dali Lama that I've always loved. He once said to a group of reporters that the proof of humanity's essentially-good nature can be seen in the daily news headlines, i.e., what is reported are the *anomalies* of human behavior, the exceptions—not the rule. Perhaps, just as the Dali Lama shifted my news-reading paradigm with that perspective, you too can counterbalance the power of a negative Tetris Effect by deciding to deliberately put a positive one into play. That is, you can use the Tetris Effect to retrain your brain so that it's programmed to scan for (and discover) the positive. If you are stressing out about things you see all around you that are going WRONG, try this SOS experiment:

First, stop your looping thoughts with a Core breath technique.

Second, dedicate a few moments to noticing what is positive around you. Focus on things that make you feel a) happy, b) grateful, or c) optimistic.

This experiment may be an effort, especially if you are trained to be vigilant for problems, or if your job is to notice all the things that need to be fixed, or if you live in a neighborhood where you have to constantly scan for real danger.

But I promise that if you find a safe, quiet place where you can do this for even a few moments, it will reduce your immediate stress and increase your sense of well being. (I especially recommend it as a "parenthesis" before and after sleeping.) Over time, you will develop the discrimination to know when and where each Tetris lens is appropriate—and you will no longer have one fixed lens with which to view our highly changeable world. *Go to Section II to learn more (p 200).*

#23: Get Inspired

(2-4 minutes)

How to do SOS #23: Inspiration means to "breathe in spirit". My experience is that inspiration connects me on a deeply personal level not only with my great colleagues and friends, but also with wonderful artists, writers, painters, philosophers, scientists, inventors, journalists, and social change agents from all times and places. When you are inspired, you connect to other great people whose ideas challenge your own beliefs or whose heroic actions urge you to do more with your life.

Here's another reason to get inspired. One of my favorite college music professors was Dominick Argento; he was widely considered America's preeminent composer of lyric opera and won the Pulitzer Prize for his song cycle, *From the Diary of Virginia Woolf.* While my thesis advisor, Dr. Argento told me something I found remarkable: that he believed there are three parties who are required to bring any composition to life: the writer of the music, the performer, and the audience. So, think of it this way: whenever you get inspired, you are participating in the enlivening of whatever work of art you have chosen.

I suggest that you mix it up. You can do this SOS exercise by taking just a few minutes a day to read a page from a great work of literature, dig into a self-help topic, learn a new phrase in a foreign language, contemplate beautiful images, listen to heart-expanding music, watch a few moments of a stimulating lecture, or read verses from the Bible, Koran, Torah or Vedas.

What's great about the SOS remedy is that we get to choose whatever sources and media we find most inspiring. And every time we do so, I we lift ourselves and others to new heights. *Go to Section II to learn more (p 201).*

#24: Time Travel (Anticipation & Memories)

(2-4 minutes)

<u>How to do SOS #24:</u> The human Mind has a very odd sense of time. Indeed, it has difficulty distinguishing between past, present and future—and experiences pretty much everything as happening NOW.

The bad news is that, under stress, our mental time travel tends to be a negative experience. Perversely, we tend to *anticipate* the worst possible outcomes and hold on to unpleasant *memories* about when things went badly for us, vividly recalling our failures, disappointments, regrets, sadness, and shame. And because the Mind is not built to distinguish clearly between now from then, we unwittingly add insult to injury by re-experiencing those tough times as if they were happening to us *right now*. Not only is this a poor use of our current time (and time travel capacity)—it makes us far less effective in the moment.

But you do have the option of directing the Mind so it travels instead to pleasant memories and a happier imagined future. That way, if you don't like your current state, you can daydream about a better one. Here's how....

Anticipation: Shift your mind from today's problem to an event you're looking forward to experiencing. If you don't have one, make one. Mark it in your calendar, so you can refer to it often. Talk to people about how excited you are about it. Find a picture of your vacation destination and make it your screen saver or put a photo on your refrigerator, where you'll see it frequently. That way you get to experience *now* the pleasure of the upcoming reality. You can also use this time-travel trick to attain a health goal, such as achieving an optimal weight.

Memories: A great way to reduce stress is relive your happy memories. When you're feeling off-balance, out-of-sorts, crabby—stop for just a moment and think back to a time when you were very happy, relaxed, having a great time. Enter that memory entirely: remember colors, sounds, smells, and the people who were there. Take a few moments to savor that wonderful moment and be grateful for it. (This is a very healthy habit to form for easing you in and out of sleep; it will replace fretting about events of the day or worrying about tomorrow.)

Here's another tip for time-traveling: If you write down your good experiences, not only will you enjoy the mental time-travel itself, but you will also strengthen the memory of its wonderful details. This works to double your fun by fully enjoying that time yet again. Use a journal or a gratitude log that you can revisit whenever you wish. *Go to Section II to learn more (p 202).*

#25: Mirror of the Mind

(6 minutes)

How to do SOS #25: This technique is a very popular exercise taught in the Silva Method. It is a powerful visualization technique that moves you from stress to success by clearly imaging what is real to you now versus what you wish for. I have listed the step-by-step instructions below, or you can go to "Learn More" for audio instructions given by Laura Silva.

Step 1. Sit quietly. Close your eyes. You can use any of the Core centering techniques to relax. Then, do the "3 to 1" countdown technique (SOS #7).

Step 2. Imagine a full-length mirror. See it as being like a movie screen that is a comfortable distance in front of you. You can make this mirror any size you want, so it is able to encompass anything or anyone you want to see within its frame.

Step 3. In your mind's eye, make the frame of this mirror a blue color. Next, project into the mirror the situation that is upsetting you. See the problem as clearly as you can, but keep it at a dispassionate distance. Take a moment to study this problem thoroughly. As you do this, you're turning the problem into a project you're going to solve. When you are done looking at this mirror image, completely erase your problem from the mirror.

Step 4. Move this cleared mirror to the left in your internal visual field, and then change the mirror's frame from blue to white. Next, create and project an image of your ideal solution into this white-framed mirror. See the solution in as much detail as you can. Feel it. Enjoy it!

Step 5. From this point forward, any time you think of this stressful situation, clearly visualize the image of your *white-framed Mirror of the Mind solution*. Recall this image as frequently as you wish. You have planted a seed in your mind. Now all you need to do is reinforce your belief that this solution is on its way. Like a real seed, it only needs time to grow. By recalling this image frequently, your happiness and belief will grow because you know that, on some level, you have already achieved your goal. *Go to Section II to learn more (p 203).*

#26: C'mon, Get Happy!

(2-4 minutes)

<u>How to do SOS #26:</u> Happiness is its own reward. When you're feeling anxious, just think instead about something that makes you happy: being with friends and family, singing, watching children play, dancing the samba, or laughing out loud. Anything. Getting happy can be as simple as deciding to turn on that mental happiness switch.

AND this activity is highly contagious. As a result of exciting research in the relatively new field of Positive Psychology, more and more people are now putting the science of happiness to pragmatic, daily use. And, in do doing, they are changing their own lives (and the lives of others) for the better.

Here's what Positive Psychology has discovered:

a) If you write down three happy things you did today, you will be significantly happier *right now*; and

b) If you make this practice a habit, your happiness will endure for a *full 6 months* beyond the time of writing. (How's that for a fantastic ROI?)

So…it's up to you. All you've got to do is make a decision to "get happy". *Go to Section II to learn more (p 204).*

#27: How Much Will this Matter in…?

(4-6 minutes)

How to do SOS #27: When you are completely entangled in a problem, here is a fast way to reframe the situation and regain some valuable perspective. Simply ask yourself: "How much will this (situation/issue/problem) matter in a…

…month? …year? …decade? …century?"

Reflect on your answers. By taking just a couple minutes to ask this quick reframing question, you can pop out of a hypnotic workaholic state—and perhaps also release any illusions you have about your own self-importance. You are also likely to gain the dispassionate judgment you need to determine whether or not this particular situation is truly an emergency.

In some cases, your answers will be: "Yes, this matters a lot because....", or "Yes, this is vital for me to do right now", etc. However, in many other instances, the answer will be: "Basta! Enough for tonight." Or, "I'll come back to this when I'm refreshed and can think straight."

The other advantage of asking yourself this question is that it could help you regain your balance by forcing you to pause long enough to remember other priorities that have slipped your mind—perhaps even ones that could have much longer positive impact. For example, getting home for dinner may have a good influence on your children in a year versus the relatively shorter impact of completing a task before you walk out the door. Another example is that decompressing so you get a good night's sleep or waking earlier to exercise could build habits that improve your health today and into the coming year and decade. *Go to Section II to learn more (p 206).*

#28: How Did You Contribute to This?

(3-4 minutes)

How to do SOS #28: This is another helpful reframing question. When we first face problems, we often have a strong urge to find out who else might be responsible—so we can blame them and/or complain to others. HOWEVER, if you ask the question "How did I contribute to this... (situation? problem? bad result?)", you assume your personal responsibility and reclaim your power to act in ways that change future outcomes.

I know that this SOS activity is not likely to be a popular stress-reducing suggestion. However it is a powerful technique because it puts you in the driver's seat. I'm not talking about assuming the blame for others, or self-berating, or putting yourself in harm's way when somebody is looking for a scapegoat. (Don't let anyone play pin-the-tail-on-the-donkey with you when you're just trying to be the adult in the group.)

This bold response is merely a way for you to learn from the situation: Here you are. You have this problem. You ask yourself: "What is my part in it? What did I do to help create it?"

The approach is powerful because if you know these answers, you'll have a better idea about how to prevent this problem from recurring. Otherwise, you're doomed to do the same thing again—and have the same undesirable outcomes repeat...and repeat. *Go to Section II to learn more (p 206).*

#29: Mental Shielding

(4-6 minutes)

How to do SOS #29: You need a good sense of humor and a willingness to play in order to do this technique. Mental shielding can be a lot of fun. The first step is to determine where you'd like to have some protection from the contagion of second-hand stress (nasty people, hostile workplace, a sociopathic boss, a crowded subway car) and then choose your personal shield. This, of course, is just an imaginary tool—but the Mind is very powerful, and I have seen many of my clients use their shields to great effect (including transforming jobs they would have left if they did not have this unusual remedy). Others have stabilized conditions so they could leave jobs on their own terms versus being pushed out. This tool also works at home: one client used it to endure time with a hostile in-law.

There is some interesting science to support Mental Shielding as a stress reduction technique. Researchers have found that people can both positively and negative affect others with their thoughts. In one study, subjects were put behind a screen or in a nearby room. The researchers then directed a group to direct negative or positive thoughts to the subject. The amazing result was that the subjects' muscle strength was significantly impacted. That is, those subjects who had positive thoughts directed at them became measurably stronger whereas those who were sent negative thoughts became measurably weaker. (Interested in trying out that shield now?)

I've listed other examples of my clients' mental shielding ideas in "Learn More" to stimulate your own thinking. All you have to do is find an image of your own that makes you feel safer, lighter, stronger, and happier. Then have a good time by playing with it. *Go to Section II to learn more (p 208).*

#30: Subliminal Stress Relief

(6 minutes)

How to do SOS #30: This is another stress relief activity where you sit back and let someone else do all the work. Just try the link below to enjoy a free sample of a sophisticated approach for reprogramming both your subconscious and conscious mind (in this case, to make you feel more healthy.)

Got to richardaluck.com/videos/check-out-this-sample-subliminal-video/ for a sample subliminal video that packs thousands of visual and auditory affirmations into just 6 minutes via "binaural and subliminal message technology". Luck claims to multiply the positive effects of traditional affirmations by using *subconscious confusion* to deliberately bypass any negative looping messages that your brain would otherwise send to occupy your mind and make your stress worse.

I have tried this cutting edge technology and think it's worth exploring. *Go to Section II to learn more (p 210).*

#31: Reframe Stress as a Friend and Teacher

(1-2 minutes)

How to do SOS #31: Mental reframing is very powerful; it also is incredibly fast acting. In fact, deciding to deliberately switch your perspective can have an almost-instant positive impact.

Reframing is NOT like taking a happy pill so you can deny real problems. A lot of people argue that we need to "face facts" – and that if we don't focus hard on fixing what's wrong we are delusion or as dangerously irresponsible as Nero fiddling while Rome burns or Scarlett O'Hara saying: "I can't think about that today. If I do, I'll go crazy. I'll think about that tomorrow."

Rather, reframing is a conscious choice, a decision to not become paralyzed by staring overly long or directly at a complex problem (a bit like looking into the eyes of the Hydra). Reframing reflects a realization that the causes of a problem may lay elsewhere, and that a fresh perspective provided by a different vantage point or extra time can make all the difference in the world to finding a lasting solution. (Indeed, Scarlett may be right that "tomorrow is another day".)

One powerful reframing approach is to think of stress as being your Ally—your new BFF, a wise teacher who has truths to tell you that will help you move from stress to success. For example, you can apply this reframing exercise in a difficult situation by asking yourself these kinds of questions:

What stimulus triggered this stressful situation?

When have I felt this stress before?

How did I respond previously (was it effective)?

How does this stress affect me/how does it make me feel?

What is this stress trying to teach me?

What positive action can I take in this moment?

When you ask questions like these, you are beginning a dialogue with your new friend (who is in a great position to offer some helpful insights). *Go to Section II to learn more (p 210).*

#32: Give Your Eyes a Break

(1-2 minutes)

How to do SOS #32: The sense that is related to the second Element of Success is, of course, Vision. Interestingly, our vision often suffers severely due to excessive stress, and eyestrain in turn contributes to further distress. Here are a few ways to give your hard-working eyes a well-deserved rest.

Option One:

Rub your palms rapidly together until they are warm. Close your eyes. Cup your palms over them. Slow your breath. (I love this one; it's so easy to do and always feels great.)

Option Two:

Remove your eyes from your computer or the papers on which you've been focused. Look at a spot far away. Keep your eyes there until they adjust to the new distance. You can also shift your eyes from a pointed single focus to look at a broad scene. When done, close your eyes for a minute of rest.

Option Three:

Unplug! Taking your eyes away from a computer screen, pad, mobile phone or TV is an excellent way to relieve eyestrain.

Your eyes (and the rest of you) will feel more rested after even a quick visual break. *Go to Section II to learn more (p 210).*

#33: Participant/Observer Dual Lens

(1-2 minutes)

How to do SOS #33: When you're feeling stressed, you could decide to put on a "dual lens" that will shift your perspective and open more choices for you. This SOS tool provides a much clearer perspective, i.e., you simultaneously act as both the Participant and the Observer. All you have to do is become internally still while in the middle of action, and then mentally step back to observe yourself while you continue to act.

This is not as hard as it sounds—and it works like magic to reduce the drama, confusion or conflict in a tough situation. It also minimizes any threat you might otherwise feel because you can switch back and forth from Participant (for example, the one who's being yelled at) to the Observer (the one who is watching actors in a film where the boss is yelling at our hero, the employee). This way you gain considerable power to act proactively rather than in a defensive knee-jerk fashion.

By participating fully in the action, you *experience events, feel your emotions, and access your intuition.* And by simultaneously observing yourself in action, you can view the situation from many different angles, thereby allowing yourself to act dispassionately and resolve the situation more creatively.

This technique is a bit like the Sounds and Silence technique (SOS #17), in that you move from foreground to background, consciously choosing your perspective in the moment.

Caveat: The power of this technique is that you retain a dual awareness. You are *simultaneously* the actor and the reviewer who is paying full attention in the audience. Stay fully involved; do NOT mentally or emotionally detach. (Checking-out by detaching is sometimes means popping out of your body; this is not the healthy, effective dual-lens response we are seeking.) *Go to Section II to learn more (p 211).*

#34: Observe, Ask, Learn, Adapt

(4-6 minutes)

<u>How to do SOS #34:</u> First Observe, then Ask, Learn, Adapt.

A. *Observe:* Where does distress show up in your body or mind? How does it affect you? What keeps you stuck? What stops you from acting to reduce this anxiety?

B. *Ask:* What has caused your distress? What triggered it? Is this stress even yours (vs. second hand stress)?

C. *Learn:* What works well, what does not, and why? Notice which of your thoughts and actions increase vs. decrease the stress you feel about this problem. Determine what you need to do differently the next time you experience a similar situation.

D. Adapt: Put what you've learned into practice. Many people contend that this sort of pragmatic practice and resulting adaptation defines the kind of intelligence that is vital for survival, evolution, and thriving both as individuals and groups.

Happily the steps in this mental process require that you learn and change accordingly. This SOS practice offers a highly effective alternative to the famous definition of insanity, i.e., doing the same thing over and over, yet expecting different results! *Go to Section II to learn more (p 211).*

Chapter Three:

Blast Through Obstacles

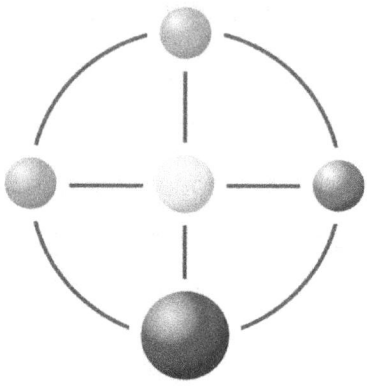

The techniques in this chapter will help you reduce stress so you become more action-oriented, disciplined, focused, and decisive; develop stronger personal boundaries; experience more ambition and drive; feel passionate about what you're doing, proud of your accomplishments, and convinced that you're making a meaningful difference; encourage you to take initiative and act assertively; make you feel more energetic.

The third Element of Success is Mission. In *The Balancing Act,* this third element corresponds to the direction of South on the wheel (see image above), the classical element of Fire, and in human beings, the personal Will. It shows up as confidence and excitement about accomplishing your burning desires.

Mission gives you definiteness of purpose. It launches you into strong action that helps you blast through obstacles. It points the way to using your special gifts and unique experiences so you can make a real difference in the world. This element propels you in the direction of your ideal Vision. It also provides the courage you'll need to get unstuck, plus the staying power you'll need to keep moving in the face of challenges.

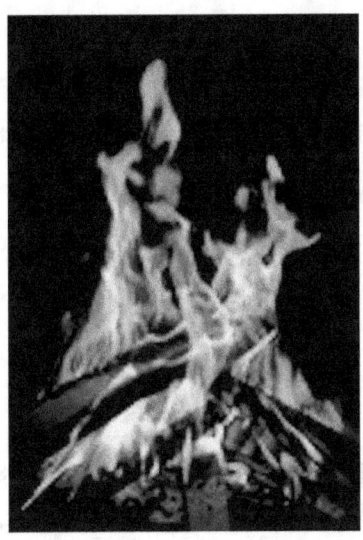

This third element of success shows up as "fire in the belly". It determines how well you set priorities and how doggedly you stay on track to achieve your goals. A strong Mission results in a can-do attitude, self-discipline, consistent behavior, a relentless never-give-up persistence, plus personal power and passion. Mission also includes motivation, dedication, focus, commitment, and the kind of initiative that flourishes when you have sufficient autonomy to do your work and the freedom you need to learn from your mistakes.

This third Element of Success also influences how assertively (vs. passively or aggressively) you handle conflict. Distress in the Mission element is likely to show up as: internal conflict among your own priorities; external conflict between your priorities and those of others; overwhelm or burn-out from the demands of having too much to do; a tendency toward procrastination; or reluctance to make decisions or act on them.

Instead of letting distress direct your behavior, the SOS techniques in this chapter will help you Stop and Think BEFORE you act. This step continues the natural order of the upward Spiral of Synergy: i.e., after you've paused and Reset from the Core, it will be easier to Reframe and think more clearly—and, as a result, you will be able to Reprioritize and act more decisively, to much greater effect.

As the third step in the TBA Change process, Mission requires you to take strong action, overcome obstacles, and do whatever is most necessary to stay on track and achieve your goals. Happily, setting a strong intention with clear priorities is much easier when your Mission is moving you closer to an ideal Vision that is rooted in your Core. *For more information on Mission, read pages 100-111 in The Balancing Act* (To read more about TBA, go to http://balance.thecoreporation.com.)

––––––––––

SOS Techniques that Blast through Obstacles:

35. Experience the Motivating Element of Mission (p 81)

36. The 5 Rites of Rejuvenation (p 82)

37. Set a Strong Intention (p 83)

38. Just Do It! (p 85)

39. Activate Your Energy (The 20-second Rule) (p 86)

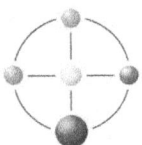

#35: Experience the Motivating Element of Mission

(2-4 minutes)

How to do SOS #35: Go to thecoreporation.com home page (or the sos_links page) and click on the Mission meditation audio. Then sit back, listen to my voice, and let me do all the work. *Go to Section II to learn more (p 213).*

#36: The 5 Rites of Rejuvenation

(6 minutes)

How to do SOS #36: The 5 Tibetan Rites of Rejuvenation is an invigorating practice that I highly recommend. There's a bit of a learning curve here, but once you get the hang of this protocol, it's quite easy and fast to do. I suggest that you start by doing a few repetitions of each exercise, and then add more as you grow stronger. You also can do any one of these techniques separately (about 1-2 minutes each) as an energizing-boosting break that's guaranteed to get you moving again.

It may take some time before you are able to build up to a full cycle of the 5 Rites. I suggest that you begin with small doses by doing only three rounds of each exercise. Soon you'll be doing 7 to 14 repetitions each, which will take only 5 or 6 minutes to complete and fit easily into your busy schedule. (The full round of 21 repetitions per rite takes 10-15 minutes to complete.) When you experience the benefits of this tool, you'll be eager to make this activity a regular part of your life.

The following videos provide easy-to-follow instructions:

- 5-minute version: (v=juZxrvc8-A4)

- Full version--15 minutes: (v=juZxrvc8-A4)

- 2-minute demo: (v=oAS9dKpML08; in Spanish).

Caution: Go easy when first learning this technique so you avoid any possibility of strain or injury. For example, the first spinning exercise may make you dizzy, so do only a few rotations until your body adjusts. Similarly, move slowly while first learning the 5 Rites so you do not overly stretch muscles in your back, arms, neck or legs. The benefit of this activity will begin right away, so you don't have to push yourself to get in the full count. *Go to Section II to learn more (p 214).*

#37: Set a Strong Intention

(6-10 seconds)

How to do SOS #37: In this SOS activity you'll learn how to do two fast *anchors* that will help you set a powerful intention. You can use these anchors for any intention: for example, to control your temper, to release fear, to access creativity for problem solving, or to quickly release stress so you can fully relax before starting a difficult meeting.

Start by sitting comfortably with your eyes closed. Bring an image of yourself to mind, for example, as already being relaxed and at ease in that upcoming meeting. Hold that image and feeling of total comfort, and then…

Option One:

…with a closed mouth, take the tip of your tongue and touch it to the roof of your mouth. Hold it there while you count up slowly from one to three. That's it.

You can touch the middle of the palate or the gum line inside your teeth; either is okay. Putting your tongue on the roof of your mouth becomes a trigger for your mind so that it comes to attention. This technique is called the *Bagha*.

Option Two:

…hold the tips of your thumb and first two fingers together for just a moment while you hold that image and feeling of being relaxed in a successful meeting. (You can use one or both hands with this anchor).

These Mission enhancing, goal-setting anchors have an added benefit. They also allow you to bring that intention back into focus at any later time when you want to strengthen your resolve. For example, if people start yelling at each other in the meeting, you can use this technique to recall your intention and calm things down so you can bring everyone back on track.

There are two other aspects of setting a powerful intention. The first is to align your personal Will with your Vision and Core. The second is to eliminate any unintended consequences and reduce the possibility of harm by including caveats such as: "This or something better" or, "Not by my Will, but Thine". These caveats underscore our realization that, when we set an intention, we don't always have full understanding of what is possible and/or best for us. They also will help you set a powerful intention while keeping you open to unanticipated better outcomes. *Go to Section II to learn more (p 214).*

#38: Just Do it!

(1-2 minutes)

How to do SOS #38: If you are feeling stuck, paralyzed by fear, frustrated or hopeless, sometimes it's a good idea simply to move. If you have no idea what to do next or any clue about how to proceed, sometimes its best to make a small decision, take a tiny action, get that feedback from the environment and move on from there.

If you want to change your life for good, it is vital that you act. And any action you take will be more effective if it's rooted in your Core values and clear Vision. So, whenever possible (and it's almost always possible), take these steps to strong action:

1. Stop. Breathe in and out deeply three times; center to contact your intuitive intelligence. (Then pause.)

2. Breathe in the memory of all the information you've gathered and all the planning you've done to date. Breathe out your fear of making a wrong decision. Do this three times. (Pause.)

3. Breathe out your decision. Write it down. (Pause.)

4. Now ACT on it. It's vital that you take one small immediate step—now. (See Activate Your Energy, SOS #39 to learn how to "Just do it!") *Go to Section II to learn more (p 215).*

#39: Activate Your Energy (The 20-Second Rule)

(20 seconds)

How to do SOS #39: If you're feeling stressed because there's some action you're not taking (a task you're avoiding, a new habit you're failing to do [eating better, exercising, etc.])—you can use this "20-second rule" to activate your energy.

Research has found that if you reduce the time it takes to initiate a task, you greatly improve your odds of both starting that task and staying with it until it forms a new habit. The 20-second rule translates into a very simple math equation:

- CONSTUCT a 20-second-plus barrier in front of a bad habit you want to stop; and/or,

- REMOVE any time barriers between you and a new good habit you want to establish.

The time from thought to action must be less than 20 seconds.

Csikszentmihalyi, the author of the classic book *Flow,* called this "activation energy", i.e., the vital initial spark you need to overcome inertia and launch a positive habit. The 20-second rule sets up a new path of least resistance to a preferred habit. It bypasses a need to always rely on grit, stamina or "will-power" to achieve your goal. And because it goes a long way to taking resistance out of the equation, the 20-second rule is a very clever practice for stress-reduction.

For example, if you want to quit smoking, then the next time you have an impulse to buy cigarettes, use the 20-second rule to buy a patch or do some quick exercises instead. To eat better foods, make a list and eat something before going to grocery store; that way you're less likely to grab bad foods as you walk up and down the grocery aisle. When you return, put healthier food choices in front of your refrigerator and less nutritious food in the bottom crisper. (See other Activation Energy ideas in Learn More.)

Have some fun; get creative. Activate your Energy to blast through obstacles in the way of your Mission, i.e., excuses or poor decisions that could otherwise impede you from achieving your desired goals. *Go to Section II to learn more (p 216).*

#40: Dance, Stomp, Drum

(4-6 minutes)

How to do SOS #40: Dancing has many health benefits: it forces you to breathe deeply, increases your flexibility, strength, endurance, and self-confidence—and is an aerobic exercise. Plus, dancing promotes a sense of wellbeing and a more positive outlook. And, it is SO much fun! Dancing and drumming, like singing, was a regular part of our ancestors' cultures and daily lives. However, as humanity has gotten more sedentary, serious, and tense, we have become more removed from these life-giving practices. We even tend to think of people who dance as "dancers" and those who drum as "drummers"— skilled artists who are somehow set apart from us. Not true.

All you have to do for this stress relieving activity is to put on some music and dance, stomp or drum. (This technique assumes you're in your own space, where you won't disturb others.) Why not have some fun? Get that blood pumping. Or, you could clean out your office or home space while dancing. You don't have to be good at dancing, just move!

You can take a break for Salsa, hip-hop, stomping, other kinds of dancing, or drumming by following along with video lessons. (I have included numerous instructional links in Learn More.) Once you've learned how to do your favorite dances you can use them for fun-filled Short Burst exercise (SOS #42). *Go to Section II to learn more (p 217).*

#41: Stand Up

(6 seconds)

How to do SOS #41: When you feel yourself getting stressed or tired, just get off your derriere and STAND UP! Too many of us are chained to our desks, phones and computers during the day, our mobile devices while commuting, or our TVs at night. It's a great stress-buster to simply unplug and stand up. And it takes so little time for such a strong return. I guarantee: once you're up, you'll feel less sluggish right away.

I advise you to mix it up: sit, stand, walk around or do short bursts of exercise. Do gentle stretches to release the kinks by putting on the speakerphone while on a conference call. You also can walk while meeting with clients and/or while "writing" (by using dictation tools).

Sitting is beginning to be recognized as a major health hazard for our era of chained-to-the-desk computer workers. Many companies have purchased adjustable standing desks for their employees, in recognition of the mounting evidence about health and productivity benefits. If you can't talk your boss into an adjustable desk or can't afford to buy one yourself, you can easily create a standing section for your desk or find another surface that can substitute as your standing desk. (I use both a bureau and my grand piano as standing desks for my laptop.)

I guarantee that if you mix it up during your workday—standing, sitting, walking, stretching even for a few minutes at a time—you'll feel much better. *Go to Section II to learn more (p 218).*

#42: Short Bursts

(4-6 minutes)

How to do SOS #42: There's a whole new school of thought about exercise. Proponents of "short burst exercise" argue that you can get great exercise value *in only 3 -10 minutes a week!* (Now, isn't this what we've all been waiting for?) I've provided a link to specific instructions and videos in Section II, but the general idea goes like this:

Stretch for one minute to warm your muscles.

Exercise INTENSELY for 30 seconds. (Flat-out, so breathless.)

Rest one minute.

Do 30 seconds of flat-out activity again.

Rest one minute.

Finish with another 30 seconds of intense activity.

(That's it!)

It is also recommended that you do this process *every other day*, for a total of 3 days per week, to optimize its impact on your health. Initial research on short burst exercise challenges all our prior assumptions about exercise, indicating that this "3 minutes a week" approach could possibly provide as much benefit as 75 minutes of vigorous workout per week or as 180 minutes of moderate exercise per week. As you can imagine, this research is causing quite a stir.

I have found that it's not always easy to walk outdoors on bad-weather days or get to exercise classes. However, doing short bursts of exercise is very easy. And, it certainly obeys the 20-second activation energy rule (SOS #39), so I actually get some great exercise done no matter how busy I am. (One caveat: Please use common sense in trying this SOS activity—it is not advisable if you have a heart condition, for example.)

Most of the short burst experiments have used stationary bikes. Although I have a bike and treadmill in my building's gym, I prefer to do short bursts of dancing (my favorite), brain gym, or jumping rope right in my home office when I feel sluggish. The options for this activity are unlimited—and it's amazing how quickly it will refresh you while the health benefits add up.

Note: A variation of this short burst workout is "high intensity training" (HIT). This is a slightly longer (10-minute) exercise format, i.e., three cycles of a 3-minute slow workout followed by 30-seconds of intermittent flat-out bursts of high-intensity activity. Again, this protocol is to be done only on alternate days. *Go to Section II to learn more (p 219).*

#43: Do One Thing

(2 minutes)

How to do SOS #43: When you feel overwhelmed with all you have to accomplish: stop, breathe, take a moment, and then select *just one thing* to do next. Refer back to your Mission, Vision and Core to determine the priorities on which you need to focus. *You need to choose.* You may have to say "no" to someone who wants your attention and it's likely you'll have to let go of other less-vital matters for the time being.

Do NOT try to multi-task—research has indicated that it will only increase your stress. Indeed, you may need to unplug from some electronic devices to focus on the main task at hand (for example, you may need to rethink the "efficiency" of texting or sending emails while on a phone call.) I think of multi-tasking as a form of cheating that comes from indecision about, and a lack of commitment to, what's most important. Multi-tasking is a way of deluding yourself that you can get everything done if you perform tasks simultaneously. (Note: Replacing SOS habits for less functional ones is *not* multi-tasking; changing the way you breathe while walking, or listening to calming music while working, will reduce your stress rather than increase it.)

I urge you to let go of the pressure of multi-tasking. To quote Lord Chesterfield (an 18th century British leader):

There is time enough for everything in the course of the day,

if you do but one thing at once,

but there is not time enough in the year,

if you will do two things at a time.

This quote reflects his belief that a singular focus was the best way to structure time *and* a sign of intelligence. He continues:

This steady and undissipated attention to one object,

is a sure mark of a superior genius;

as hurry, bustle, and agitation,

are the never-failing symptoms of a weak and frivolous mind.

I have long thought of multi-tasking as an illusory concept that has done all of us a great disservice. As it now turns out, science agrees with me! Multi-tasking was an attempt by humans to mimic computers' abilities. In truth, we now know that the human brain can focus on just one thought at a time. So, multi-tasking only succeeds in exhausting us while confusing our priorities and derailing our best efforts. Not to mention, it makes us feel inadequate because we've been told that really smart people can multi-task brilliantly. What a crock!

Some people believe we'll eventually be able to train the human brain so it's better at multi-tasking. But until then, I recommend that you follow the sage advice that Jack Palance's character gave Billy Crystal's character in the 1991 movie *City Slickers*: The "Secret of Life…", the cowboy Curley revealed, "…is to do One Thing." *Go to Section II to learn more (p 220).*

#44: Shake it, Baby, Shake it!

(2 minutes)

How to do SOS #44: Stand up. Put your feet firmly on the ground, hip's distance apart. Start by shaking both your hands (gently) at the wrist. Then shake your arms, all the way up to your shoulders. Next shake your head and neck (gently) while continuing to shake your arms. Now you're ready to shake your trunk—shoulders, chest, and hips. Shake it, Baby, Shake it!

And now let your legs join in, lifting one at time and shaking it fully. Lastly, let both your feet move while you continue to shake your whole body. Move around the room, shaking your body. (Don't go crazy here and throw anything out of joint; just keep shaking your body gently until it feels loose and happy.)

Do this "Shake-it" whole-body exercise for two minutes, from start to finish. Then stand straight again, feet firmly planted, drawing yourself up as tall as you can. Pause while breathing deeply in and out. Notice that all your body's stressful contracting is gone. Feel the blood pumping—doesn't it feel great? Allow your breath to slow and return to normal, and then go on with your day. *Go to Section II to learn more (p 221).*

#45: Change, Accept or Leave

(4-6 minutes)

How to do SOS #45: If you are having a hard time making a decision, this approach could help you break through. Perhaps it feels as if none of your options are good ones. However, the longer you avoid making a choice: the more stress you'll experience; the fewer options you'll have as time passes; and, the more likely it will be that the decision is made for you. The truth is, you only ever have three distinct choices: 1) You can change the situation, and if that is not possible, 2) you will have to accept it, or 3) you will need to leave it.

So…ask the following questions to help you make the best possible decision among these three options:

What in this situation is possible for me to change?

Am I willing to exert the effort necessary to make this change?

When am I likely to know if this change is going to work?

And if change is not going to work, which is better for me to do: accept that reality or leave—and why?

To support you in making a good decision (and/or sticking to it once it's made), consider using the famous serenity prayer: "God grant me the serenity to accept the things I cannot change; Courage to change the things I can; and Wisdom to know the difference." *Go to Section II to learn more (p 222).*

#46: Never Fail

(2-4 minutes)

How to do SOS #46: The fear of failure is highly stressful and often paralyses us into inaction, procrastination, and a sense of overwhelm. Tim Phizackerley of PSTEC fame (see SOS #54) has a brilliant technique that reduces stress by increasing your confidence so you will never have to fail again.

The idea is simple. He suggests that instead of rating your success or failure on other people's reactions to your actions, *you rate YOUR success or failure on whether or not you acted.* It's a revolutionary idea—and a highly pragmatic one. Clearly, we can control only our own behavior, and never anyone else's action or reaction. And it is *always* within our power to act.

So...the next time you decide to pick up the phone to call a potential client, you can declare the very fact that you took action to be a success and celebrate it, independent of that person's response. The good news, of course, is that you are increasing your odds of success because you will act more confidently and energetically. This makes you more appealing when you finally do make that call you've been avoiding.

By reframing "failure" and "success" in this new action-oriented way, you're more likely to catapult yourself out of being stuck. Additionally, you'll be happier because you'll have more daily experiences of success that you can build on to create even greater successes. *Go to Section II to learn more (p 223).*

#47: Reduce Resistance

(2-4 minutes)

How to do SOS #47: Your own internal resistance can cause considerable stress and discomfort. If you're having an internal debate about whether or not to do something, you will experience resistance. However, this resistance can be instructive: ask yourself what the internal conflict is about—and, how should you act: a) now, and b) in the future to address the roots of it?

If you have unpleasant feelings you're trying to push down and/or ignore, sometimes it's better to release them in safe ways. Similarly, if you have a task you must accomplish, it can require more energy to *avoid* doing it rather than just doing it. (See SOS #53 and SOS #54 for fast-acting emotional release techniques. These two SOS tools reduce the resistance of emotional blocks that prevent, rather than allow, what you DO desire from coming into your life.)

Resistance is another name for your good friend, Stress. Sometimes resistance can be a friend that urges you to say no to people who are demanding your time and attention for their (vs. your) agenda. You can reduce your resistance in this case by determining how their demands fit within your Mission. This careful response will go a long way to strengthening your personal boundaries so you become increasingly clear about what you will and will not do. It also will decrease the number of unrealistic requests and inappropriate demands on your time.

So…when you feel resistance, listen to it. Then you'll be able to make good choices that support your Mission, Vision and Core. *Go to Section II to learn more (p 223).*

#48: Power Poses

(2 minutes)

How to do SOS #48: Power poses are terrific *two-for-the-price-of-one* activities—they simultaneously decrease your stress AND increase your confidence. Standing in a power pose for *only two minutes* can change your sense of self-motivation and make you more willing to act decisively. Examples of power poses include: the "Super Woman/Superman" pose (hands on hips with feet apart, head held high); the crossing-the-finish-line "victory" pose (hands thrown up in the air); and the confident executive pose (hands linked behind your head, with feet up on your desk). See Amy Cuddy demonstrate at ted.com/talks/amy_cuddy_your_body_language_shapes_who_you_are.

These poses may sound silly, but they work like a charm. Just DO them! Your body chemistry will change dramatically. This is an example of "faking it" until you actually become it. I have used power poses with many clients (ranging from at-risk youth to out-of-work executives to business leaders to highly anxious ex-prisoners). As a result, I can testify not only to their efficacy, but also to how much fun they are.

Researchers who had people do these poses *prior to* interviews found that these subjects not only reported feeling more confident, but also were judged more capable by those who interviewed them. Conversely, those less-fortunate control subjects who held disempowering poses before the interview (slumping, head downcast, being deferential) were judged as not being nearly as capable, intelligent, etc. Other disempowering poses include contracting positions that make your body somewhat smaller (such as crossing your legs, holding your arms over chest, etc.)

Power poses work their magic by releasing body-to-mind to hormonal signals that make people feel more assertive, confident, optimistic, willing to take risks—and amazingly, a lot *less stressed*. (What's not to love?) And, if you want to ratchet up your positive results even further, add a smile to your power pose. (See SOS #58.) *Go to Section II to learn more (p 224).*

#49: Choose Your Weapon (Conflict Style)

(4-5 minutes)

How to do SOS #49: Sometimes you just have to fight. In fact, the stress you're feeling may be because you've been trying to avoid trouble by being overly accommodating. In that case, you need to switch to becoming a "wise warrior" who carefully chooses the right weapon. By this, I mean that you need to decide what conflict management approach is most likely to work in any given situation.

Note to parents and teachers: Please consider discussing this SOS technique with your children to protect them from being victims or perpetrators of bullying. Learning a variety of conflict management skills can protect youth from both the immediate impact and long-term adverse health effects of bullying.

There are 5 basic conflict management styles: avoidance, accommodation, competition, compromise, and collaboration. To determine the best approach for your particular situation, read the definitions below; then decide upon the "weapon" you think will work best for you.

Each way of managing conflict has both advantages and disadvantages, and each is appropriate at different times (see Learn More to discover your dominant conflict management style). After you've chosen your weapon from the below list, you will be better equipped to move into strong action.

1. *Avoiding* conflict includes withdrawing from problems or suppressing differences. It might take the form of diplomatically sidestepping an issue, postponing an issue until a better time, or simply withdrawing from a threatening situation. It could also include less functional behaviors such as indifference, resignation, and surrender.

2. *Accommodating* could mean that you're neglecting your own concerns to satisfy other peoples' needs. This style may involve obeying orders when you would prefer not to, denying or avoiding differences, or yielding to others' points of view.

3. *Competing.* In this conflict style, winning provides a sense of pride and achievement. In order to "win" you may simply show some backbone by standing up for your rights—or you may "win" by exerting pressure so others capitulate to your goals.

4. *Compromise.* This style is likely to require that all parties give up something to create a mutually acceptable situation. You may need to sacrifice part of your goals to find a solution that splits the differences and exchanges concessions fairly.

5. *Collaboration.* This style recognizes all interests as a way to work creatively toward mutual gain. Although this style tends to be more time-consuming, it assumes that all parties involved *must* get their needs met to some degree for an equal, fair, sustainable outcome. *Go to Section II to learn more (p 225).*

#50: Now Power

(2-4 minutes)

How to do SOS #50: A very fast way to eliminate stress is to use a technique I learned from the *Power of Now* by Eckhart Tolle. It's so simple and portable that both my clients and I can do it just about anywhere, anytime.

All you have to do is get quiet for a moment. Use one of the Core SOS practices to do so. Then, ask yourself this question:

"What is wrong with THIS moment, right now?" (Not any moment in the past; not any potential future moment. Just focus all your attention on NOW.)

Continue to sit quietly. Continue to breathe. And continue to look—hard—for what's wrong with this moment. When you mind wanders, bring your attention to this moment.

After a few minutes of this activity, stop.

The truth is most likely to be somewhat surprising: what most people experience is that *this moment*—stripped of its past and future brackets—is just fine. *Nothing at all is wrong with it.*

If you focus on NOW, that elusive, constantly moving point in time, you will discover that it is absolutely perfect, just as it is. (This is a wonderful experience *and* an effective technique to ease you into or out of a great night's sleep.) "Now-power" will strip away all your worries, leaving you feeling great. Enjoy!

Go to Section II to learn more (p 225).

#51: Respect Your Desires

(5-6 minutes)

How to do SOS #51: It can be stressful to not have what you desire. Desires show up as impulses, point to resources we need if we're to achieve our goals—or they can flash as envy of what others have, and can even become compulsions or addictions.

The goal of this SOS technique is to reduce your stress by first, recognizing the desires you have, and then distinguishing those desires that most deserve your respect, i.e., those that could contribute to your lasting happiness and success. These desires reflect the needs of your best self. As Napoleon Hill emphasized in *Think and Grow Rich*, a "burning desire" is vital to your happiness, the accumulation of wealth, achieving your life purpose, and contributing your gifts to the world.

Step 1. Write a wish list of *everything* you desire. Take a couple minutes to brainstorm. When done, read through the whole list. If you forgot anything, write it down now.

Step 2. Set priorities in this list of what you most want. Flag desires that are most likely to result in real happiness—i.e., those that are most aligned with your Core, Vision, Mission.

(Note: If you still desire something "nonessential", see if it might actually be part of your personal or artistic expression, e.g., this work of art or that book may feed your soul and mind.)

The objective of this exercise is to be discerning so you can treat the desires you feel with the respect they deserve, as potential signals that reveal what is in your heart.

To sort out the wheat from the chaff, you can ask yourself: *Why does this matter so much to me? Why does not having it cause me stress? What do I really want? What is the desire below this desire?* (For example, "I want a million dollars" may have the underlying desire of: "I want to make sure my family is safe and well cared for.") *Go to Section II to learn more (p 226).*

Chapter Four:

Improve Emotional Intelligence

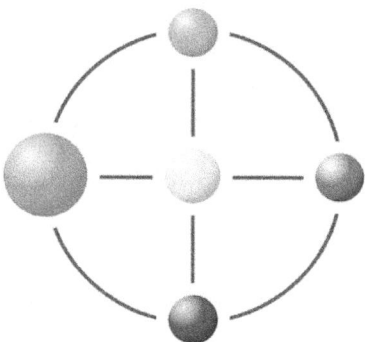

The techniques in this chapter will help you reduce stress so you: develop more healthy and supportive relationships; increase emotional stability and maturity; interact more skillfully with others; choose supportive friends and colleagues; improve communication skills; become more compassionate, respectful, loving, and caring; and expand your communities.

This fourth element of Interactions corresponds in *The Balancing Act* to the direction of West (see image above), the classical element of Water, and in human beings, the Emotions that flow between or inside us. The health of this element shows up as kindness, empathy, understanding, and strong connections with others. When you're feeling distress in this element, it's likely to be from relationship problems, emotional upheavals, "negative" feelings, or second-hand stress. In fact, your own (and others') stress can adversely affect both internal and external Interactions (interpersonal and intrapersonal).

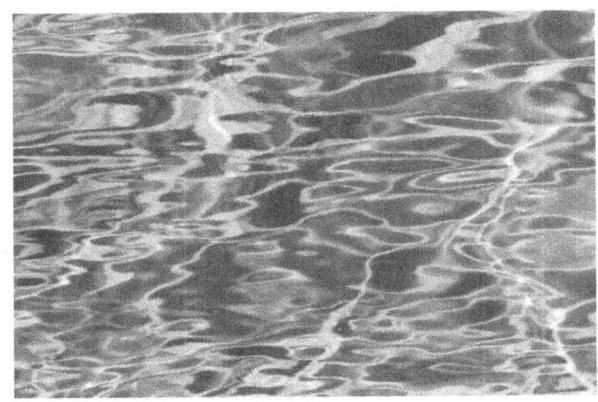

The fourth element translates into emotional intelligence (EQ). It lets you know whether or not the people around you and the situations you're experiencing are safe and healthy. (Your Core intuition passes this information on via "good" or "bad" feelings.) Often we feel that something is wrong long before our cognition kicks in and we are able to make sense of those feelings. Emotions will tell you whether you're on track toward your goals (you feel optimistic, enthusiastic, happy) or off course (you feel discomfort, fear, depression, sadness, anger).

The element of Interactions governs the happiness of your working and personal relationships, your communication skills, and how isolated or connected you feel (i.e., the strength of your family/community). It helps you shift from the strife of competition into joining forces with like-minded people so you can work together to create something worthwhile instead.

Instead of letting distress ruin your relationships or allow your emotions to run wild, you can use the SOS techniques in this chapter to continue the upward evolutionary Spiral of Success; i.e., first stopping so you can Reset from the Core, then

Reframing and directing your thoughts, and then controlling your actions and setting your priorities. This will make it more likely that your emotions and relationships are powerfully aligned with the other Elements of Success.

In the TBA Change process, the fourth step is "Relate". At this stage you will be better able to distinguish between relationships that are helpful and healthy versus those that are detrimental to your evolution, happiness, and success. (To use a colloquialism: You can't fly like an eagle if turkeys surround you.) At this step in the change process, you'll need to candidly assess who drags you down versus who helps you to soar. *For more information on Interactions, read pages 131-142 in The Balancing Act.* (To read about more about TBA or to purchase it, go to http://balance.thecoreporation.com.)

SOS Techniques that Develop Emotional intelligence:

52. Experience Compassionate Element of Interactions (p 107)
53. Transform Negative Emotions (EFT) (p 107)
54. PSTEC (Percussive Suggestion Technique) (p 109)
55. Tend and Befriend (p 110)
56. Get Over Yourself (p 112)
57. Small Acts of Kindness (p 113)
58. Smile (p 114)
59. Smile at Three Extra People (p 115)
60. Try Laughter Yoga (p 117)
61. Find a Choir to Join (p 118)

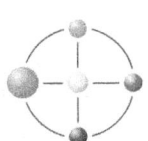

#52: Experience Compassionate Element of Interactions

(6 minutes)

How to do SOS #52: Go to thecoreporation.com home page (or the sos_links page) and click on the Interactions meditation audio. Then sit back, listen to my voice, and let me do all the work. *Go to Section II to learn more (p 227).*

#53: Transform Negative Emotions (EFT)

(4-6 minutes)

How to do SOS #53: Many emotions we consider "negative" can actually help us, i.e., they can teach us important things about ourselves (like our dear friend, Stress). This SOS technique assumes that while "negative" emotions can be overwhelming, they are best treated as raw energy that you can transform into something more useful for your evolution. As you know from observing them, emotions do change—coming and going like waves on the ocean. What you can do with this SOS tool is to befriend the full range of your emotions so all of them can help you grow.

I highly recommend the Emotional Freedom Technique (EFT), a very simple and portable process, as a great way to learn from and release "bad" feelings. EFT was developed 25 years ago by psychologist Roger Callahan (he calls it TFT or *Thought Field Therapy*) and refined later by Gary Craig (a performance engineer). In ensuing years, many others contributed to the development, simplification, broadcasting and mounting research about the efficacy of this powerful tool. EFT will serve you by quickly mutating fear, anger, anxiety, procrastination, and overwhelm into calmness and renewed energy. To experiment with EFT, simply go to the videos noted below.

There are many schools of thought about how to do EFT; just adopt whichever most appeals to you. This process involves tapping lightly on a series of acupuncture meridian points while making statements to release any negativity you're feeling. (Practitioners believe EFT "rewires" patterns in our hydraulic-based nervous system, which runs our thoughts and feelings.)

To start this activity, you will do a few rounds of statements that serve to first surface and then release the negativity you're experiencing. The second phase of EFT is to replace those statements with positive or neutral declarations.

The common points for tapping are: side of hands, top of head, inner eyebrow, side of eye, below eyes, under nose, under mouth, collar bone, under arm. There are many variations of EFT; simply choose one that's easy for you and try it out.

- A fun introduction (4 minutes; v=X4EDgTc0AyQ)

- Stress and anxiety #1 (4 minutes; v=SDGQa-9dhTk)

- Stress and anxiety #2 (5-6 minutes; v=zxk7cVPEOXw)

- See RogerCallahan.com for free TFT guide and videos.

Go to Section II to learn more (p 228).

#54: Percussive Suggestion Technique (PSTEC)

(6 minutes--or longer if you wish)

How to do SOS #54: Percussive Suggestion Technique (PSTEC), a relatively recent invention of Tim Phizackerley, is a powerful SOS technique. All you have to do to start this process is go to pstec.org for free PSTEC audio tracks (you will find them at the bottom of home page). Just follow the instructions on the sound track to do this activity. It couldn't be easier. The click tracks are about 10 minutes long, but I've included them in this book because it is easy to stop after 6 minutes if that's all the time you have available—and you will get a great return from those six minutes of using PSTEC for emotional transformation.

I want to give you the heads-up that, at first, PSTEC may feel as frustrating as simultaneously patting your head and rubbing your stomach. This however is its genius; i.e., PSTEC audio technology scrambles and releases emotionally toxic stress patterns to make way for healthier responses. The bottom line is that this unusual process really works. It has been used by thousands of people to heal their fears, stress, phobias, PTSD, anxiety, resentment, compulsions, depression, etc.

My experience with clients and myself is that PSTEC can help heal severe stress caused by negative feelings and past events such as abuse, trauma, bullying, or the specter of any prior failures repeating. PSTEC is a bit like EFT on steroids (see SOS #53). I use this technique whenever I have something that *really* upsets me and for which I need immediate emotional release. *Go to Section II to learn more (p 230).*

#55: Tend and Befriend

(3-4 minutes)

<u>How to do SOS #55:</u> One of the greatest stress relievers known to humanity is to care for and spend time with people you love. Indeed "tending and befriending" is a major alternative to the "fight or flight" stress response. Interestingly, both of these stress-responses are seen throughout the animal kingdom.

Tending is when you do nurturing activities, such as caring for offspring or someone who is injured: protecting them, feeding

110

them, ensuring their safety and wellbeing, and reducing their build-up of toxic stress. *Befriending* is when you create and maintain friendships, forming social networks that perform many of the same functions as tending. Neuroendocrine evidence from animal and human studies suggests that oxytocin and reproductive hormones may be at the core of this powerful alternate response to reducing distress.

Here are some ways *tending* works as an SOS activity. Let's say you get home from work, and then put your concerns aside for just a few moments as you listen attentively to your children's excited stories from the day. (*Poof!* Your stress is gone.) *Befriending* relieves your stress similarly, for example, when you reach out to be with good friends and/or members of your personal, professional or social communities. It only takes a few minutes to pick up the phone, text or email a friend or family member. You can also drop by a favorite colleague's desk or a neighbor's home and arrange to meet for lunch, coffee, or a healthy walk. (Again, *poof*—your stress is gone.)

Tending and befriending can be used to help you build and expand strong communities—whether extended family, professional, neighborhood, national, or world. Tending and befriending reduce not only your own, but also other peoples' stress from social isolation. And social isolation, as we're now learning, is a major health hazard; indeed, the health risks from loneliness are greater than those from smoking or obesity!

A meta-analysis of 148 studies showed that strong social systems provide a 50% greater likelihood of survival from medical problems! This phenomenon was consistent across age, gender, pre-existing conditions and other health factors. As it turns out, tending and befriending are great survival tools. *Go to Section II to learn more (p 231).*

#56: Get Over Yourself

(2- 4 minutes)

How to do SOS #56: The pain of distress can bring out the self-absorbed narcissist in any of us and contribute to our self-isolation. Unfortunately, when we focus on our own anxiety and pain, it magnifies rather than diminishes in intensity. At these times you could use this SOS technique of "getting over yourself"—here's a few ways to do so.

For starters, you can put your own troubles into a more realistic perspective by reading the news. After a few headlines about natural and political disasters, you'll see how small your problems are in comparison. You could also walk down the street or sit quietly and watch people's faces; you'll soon recognize that suffering is all around you, everyone has problems, and pain is a common part of the human experience.

The point of this tool is to urge you to make a conscious choice to feel better right now. (See SOS #19 to "Stop It!") Make a healthy decision to NOT add further to your own and everyone else's misery by dwelling overly long on your problems. Don't make your life a soap opera, with yourself in the starring role of victim. Get over it. Write another script for yourself—decide to become an "angel" for someone who really needs a helping hand, or cast yourself in a new role as hero of your own story. (See a variety of heroic archetypes in *Working from Your Core*.) *Go to Section II to learn more (p 232).*

#57: Small Acts of Kindness

(1-2 minutes)

How to do SOS #57: If you're feeling overly stressed, refocus completely by doing a small, conscious (even random) act of kindness for someone else. Train your attention on someone else's needs rather than your own. For example, you could make a call to your aunt, or go online and contribute to a natural disaster relief effort, sign up for a fundraising walk, or check in on a friend who's been having difficulty, just to see how he's doing today. There are thousands of small acts of kindness readily available to you. If you take just a couple minutes to do one small kind thing, I promise you'll feel great.

If you really want to have some fun, pay the toll for the next person in line, compliment someone who's feeling down, bring good food to a friend who's recovering from an injury, or slow down for a few minutes to talk with a neighbor. Your stress will vanish, you'll feel warm all over—and the recipient will feel great too. You may even launch a chain reaction of kindness with this one, small act. *Go to Section II to learn more (p 234).*

#58: Smile

(<6 seconds)

How to do SOS #58: Really, now—I don't have to explain how to do this, do I? Smiling is a fantastic SOS technique because it positively changes your body chemistry within seconds.

Here's how it works: When the smiling muscles in your face contract, they automatically send signals to your brain that reinforce your good feelings. Then, because your brain feels good, it signals you to smile—setting up a self-reinforcing positive loop. In next-to-no time, smiling stimulates your brain's reward mechanisms in a way that even chocolate can't match! In fact, smiling produces the same happiness rewards as exercising. Smiling not only relieves stress, it also boosts the immune system, lowers blood pressure, releases natural pain killers, contributes to long life—and makes people look younger and more attractive. (Are you smiling yet?)

And even more interestingly, your brain *keeps track* of your smiles, a bit like a smile scorecard. This way the brain knows how often you've smiled and therefore, the overall emotional state in which you live. This internal smile scorecard provides one fascinating reason why we all tend to feel happier around children: on average, they smile *400 times a day!* Even relatively happy adults smile only 40-50 times a day. (Sad to say, the average adult smiles a mere *20 times a day*.)

So…when you consider that smiling leads to a decrease in the stress-induced hormones that negatively affect many aspects of overall physical and mental health, you might want to consider smiling now and often—not only for your sake but also to benefit all those around you.

Another interesting fact about smiling: you don't have to mean it when you smile! I'm not recommending that you "fake" a smile; rather, just remember that your brain responds positively to the facial changes that constitute a smile. Try this: If you put a pencil length-wise in your mouth and hold it lightly between your teeth, you will trick your brain into thinking you're smiling—and it will provide you with many of the same health benefits as a real smile. *Go to Section II to learn more (p 235).*

#59: Smile at Three Extra People

(20 seconds)

How to do SOS #59: I do realize that it sometimes takes a concerted effort to smile. But there are so many benefits to be gained, I urge you to try. Each time you smile at another person, their brain coaxes them to return the favor. You are creating a symbiotic relationship that allows both of you to release feel good chemicals in your brain, activate reward centers, make each of you more attractive, and increase the chances that you'll both live longer, healthier lives.

Just remember: even if you are in the middle of an actual life-and-death crisis, a soft smile is a kindness that can help both for you and those around you. As Mother Teresa stated: "We shall never know all the good that a simple smile can do." Think of it your smile as a gift for anyone who is feeling distress.

This smiling activity "ups-the-ante" on the simple smile technique (SOS #58) by challenging you to smile at three more people than you might normally do today. As the old song says: "Spread sunshine all over the place, just put on a happy face." This is one of my favorite SOS tools: when I go on my daily walks, I smile at mothers and babies, neighbors, strangers (as long as they're not TOO strange and/or likely misinterpret a smile). When I go into my local shops, I smile at the beleaguered clerks and servers, who usually smile back and seem buoyed up in for the next person in line. Not only does this help others, I've noticed that these same people often greet me with a big smile when I next walk in their door (thereby returning my smile to me when I need a pick-me-up).

Frankly, this stress-reducing technique is a lot of fun. Smiling at others creates a *positive mirror contagion* (i.e., "second-hand smiling.") Research indicates that humans are wired to smile back at someone who smiles at them—which positively changes THEIR chemistry too.

Here are some caveats for you to consider with this technique:

1. Do not *expect* people to smile back. They may be having a rough day or distrust smiling strangers. Just

offer a smile with no expectation. It will still positively affect both your and their brain chemistry.

2. Make certain that your smile is not mistaken for "Hey, Sailor!" or "I'm from out of town; please mug me."

3. Be sensitive to cultural differences. Smiling is not the social norm in many countries.

These caveats should minimize any misunderstandings. *Go to Section II to learn more (p 236)*

#60: Try Laughter Yoga

(6 minutes or longer if you wish)

How to do SOS #60: The healing effects of laughter have long been known, but now there is an international movement called "Laughter Yoga", which was launched in 1995 by Madan Kataria, an M.D. from Mumbai, India. If you want to reduce your stress, you've got to check it out; just visit http://laughteryoga.org for many resources and/or listen to this terrific TED talk by Katrina with specific instructions for how to do Laughter Yoga (feature=player_embedded&v=5hf2umYC). Here is one very easy technique to get you launched:

1. Clap hands together with palms flat, fingers touching.

2. Clap to this rhythm: 1 – 2 – (then half-beats) 1-2-3.

3. Add out-loud laughter to the clapping beat: Ho – Ho – Hah-Hah-Hah.

Repeat and repeat. It's SO easy. Notice how much better your body feels after just a few minutes.

I think Laughter Yoga is a remarkable invention; it combines powerful breathing and classic yoga techniques with sustained laughter. It does NOT rely on jokes, humor, or puns to generate laughter. (These typically cause only short bursts of laughter.) In contrast, Laughter Yoga has been designed to provide the body, mind, emotions and spirit with a wonderful exercise workout. If you like this activity, you can check out the growing communities of like-minded people who help each other laugh whenever they get together. At the time of this writing there are 16,000+ Laughter Clubs in 72 countries. Kataria refers to these as the happiest communities in the world. I have no doubt he's right. *Go to Section II to learn more (p 237).*

#61: Find a Choir to Join

(5-6 minutes)

How to do SOS #61: Of all types of singing, it's *choral singing* that most multiplies the health benefits of singing (see SOS #9). Research indicates that choral singing has a major positive impact on people's lives: those who sing in choirs have greater life satisfaction, plus significantly less depression and anxiety. Indicators are that group singing also reduces pain, increases memory, and improves self-esteem.

All you have to do in this SOS activity is take a few minutes to explore: Do a computer search for local choirs, ask a friend, or talk to a minister. Just find a choir that seems appealing to you—look for the kind of music you enjoy, people who seem to be fun, a practice schedule that's doable, and a place that's reasonably easy to get to.

That's the extent of this SOS technique: just find a choir. Later, you'll need to take some time to check out the possibilities you've turned up—then sign up for the one you most like. Once you do find that choir, *each one of the choral songs you practice will be a powerful, fast SOS technique for that day.*

Happily, you don't need a great voice to join many choirs—you just have to be willing to lend your voice to a group that suits you. Singing in a choir is a great community builder that creates happiness for you, your singing buddies, and all the people who come to hear you. *Go to Section II to learn more (p 239).*

#62: Loving Kindness

(1 minute and 4 minute variations)

How to do SOS #62: This is a loving affirmation and blessing that is common to the Buddhist, Christian and Jewish traditions. Here is the first variation I learned; it includes yourself, and may be a good place to start when you're feeling overly stressed.

Option One:

May I be safe; May I be happy;

May I be healthy; May I live with ease.

May you be safe….

May we be safe….

Option Two:

A longer variation of this beautiful blessing directs loving kindness to a variety of people, according to the following list. As you say each person's name, visualize and send love to him or her, repeating the below script three times each:

May you be well. May you be happy.

May you be peaceful. May you be loved.

#1. Send loving kindness to someone you respect or admire.

#2. Someone you love (a child, mate or family member).

#3. A neutral person (an acquaintance or a clerk at a shop).

#4. Someone you dislike or with whom you're having difficulty.

By sending loving-kindness in this order, you will systematically break down the barriers between yourself and these four types of people in your life. *Go to Section II to learn more (p 240).*

#63: Green—Yellow—Red Light

(2-4 minutes)

<u>How to do SOS #63:</u> One of the easiest ways I know to help people access their emotional GPS intelligence is by having them ask the "Green light–Yellow light–Red light" question. You

can use this with people about whom you're unsure. Your internal GPS will give you an answer via your feelings. All you have to ask is: *Do I feel good (green light) or undecided (yellow light) or bad/yucky/confused (red light) around this person?*

Listen to the "gut" response from your emotional guidance system. Pay attention; these are survival signals upon which you should rely. Once you're aware of how you really feel, you'll be able to make intelligent working decisions about how you interact with everyone. This technique can be a lifesaver.

When you listen for an answer, just pay attention to how you FEEL: Does this person make you feel happy? Increase or lessen your stress? Make you feel more or less good about yourself? Do you have any instinctive misgivings about this person? Is what this person says congruent with what s/he does? Do you feel thrown off-balance or more centered? How much trust do you experience around him or her?

A caveat: Proceed with caution at the start of using this activity. Many people have had their emotional GPS damaged during childhood. If this is true for you, just practice until your innate GPS recalibrates and you can feel that it is doing its natural job for you. *Go to Section II to learn more (p 241).*

#64: Give (and Get) a Hug

(30 seconds)

How to do SOS #64: To start, use this activity only with people you know well. The beauty of a hug is that BOTH people have their stress relieved! The underlying reason a hug works so well to relieve stress is that, within 20 seconds, a hug releases oxytocin. This is sometimes called the "feel-the-love" hormone, and its positive effects include decreasing anxiety, increasing a sense of satisfaction with life, and helping human beings feel bonded. With a hug we remind ourselves of our affection and break down the barriers between us.

A few caveats: 1. Take care to respect others' boundaries; some people love hugging, yet others find such familiarity offensive; 2. Make certain the hug is in no way improper or sexual; and, 3. Be sensitive to cultural differences (some cultures are much more "okay" with touching than others).

All that being said, hugging is a great way to break the invisible bubble of distress that keeps us separate when we could be reaching out to offer care and help instead. As Virginia Satir, a respected family therapist states: "We need four hugs a day for survival. We need eight hugs a day for maintenance. We need twelve hugs a day for growth."

So…go out there and get those 8-12 hugs a day! (Just choose your "hugees" carefully so you don't become a "mad-hugger" from whom people flee.) *Go to Section II to learn more (p 242).*

#65: Say Thank You

(1-2 minutes)

How to do SOS #65: This is a very fast SOS technique that has countless benefits. All you have to do is to think of someone you should thank for something–almost anything. Then you could: send that person an email, or call them, or walk out the office door and say something that shows your appreciation for them. You could also thank your waiter for service, your bus/cab driver, or the clerk at the counter. They will feel good— and you'll feel good. Also, it's the right thing to do.

Truth is, we don't thank the people around us as often as they deserve to be thanked. If you thank people in your workplace, they will consider it a sign of respect. You'll likely notice improved morale and more willingness to cooperate as a result. And if you do this at home, your family will feel more noticed and appreciated; it also is great behavior to model for your children so they learn how to do this at a very early age.

So start spreading gratitude among people you know in this simple, direct, easy way. *Go to Section II to learn more (p 242).*

#66: Reversal Tapping

(1 minute)

How to do SOS #66: This is a fast and easy SOS technique that has many of the benefits of EFT (SOS #53). Here's how to do it: repeatedly tap the Karate chop points of both hands together (these are the fleshy outsides of your hands) while repeating a script that relates to the issue troubling you:

"I deeply and completely love myself, accept myself, respect myself, and appreciate myself, even though...*I have trouble letting go of my worries about money.... Or I'm having difficulty releasing my anger at Susan.... Or I can't let go of my fear about this meeting with my boss."* Repeat three times. Done.

And here's a variation of reversal tapping that supposedly ratchets up the degree of emotional release and speeds results: On each hand, touch the tips of your thumbs to your fourth ("ring") finger. Then proceed with the karate chop and script as noted above. *Go to Section II to learn more (p 243).*

#67: Connect with a Critter

(2-4 minutes)

How to do SOS #67: There's hardly a better coping mechanism known to humanity than connecting with our friends in the animal kingdom (many of whom seem to have their own stress under much better control than we do).

Animals are so effective at calming people down that they are used with increasing frequency for healing PTSD for returning soldiers and survivors of natural disasters or terrorist attacks. There are also strong indicators that contact with animals can speed surgical recovery and reduce isolation, which is why some hospitals and rest homes have instituted pet programs.

My brother Tom and nephews Aidan and Kieren used to bring their loveable Bassett hound, Garth, to the neighborhood rest home. He was such a hit that I dubbed him Garth-the-Healer.

If you don't have a pet of your own, you can still do this activity. Just find a happy-to-see-you dog in your neighborhood or hold a willing cat in your lap until it purrs (of course, with permission of both the animals and their owners). And although actual physical contact seems to bring the most health benefits, you can also reduce stress by observing fish swimming languidly in a tank or watching wild creatures in their natural habitat. Need I go on? *Go to Section II to learn more (p 244).*

#68: What Are You Feeling?

(20 seconds)

How to do SOS #68: A fast way to increase your emotional intelligence is to become aware of what you're feeling in any given moment. Often people are out-of-touch with their emotions. We actually don't really know how we feel—and that is a real handicap to managing stress. The good news is: if you can improve your ability to quickly understand what you're feeling, you will be able to stop distress earlier in the cycle, i.e., before it has advanced to the "red flag" of physical symptoms or turned the corner into disease. (See SOS #74.)

A way I've used to help clients increase their EQ is to have them set their watch or phone timer for regular emotional-intelligence check-ins. It's easy: Whenever the buzzer goes off, just stop and ask yourself: What emotion am I feeling right now? Write it down. This takes less than 20 seconds.

This is one way to start taking control of your emotional health. And, just in case you're new to this, you can use the below list of emotions as a place to begin. Circle the emotion you're feeling or write it in your EQ check-in log.

Emotions are said to fall into the following four main categories. This list is not comprehensive, so feel free to add other emotions as you experience them.

Glad: Love, Appreciation, Gratitude, Passion, Affection, Care; Joy, Optimism, Hopefulness; Happiness, Contentment, Satisfaction, Security; Empowerment, Freedom; Trust, Respect, Acceptance
Sad: Depression, Melancholy; Nostalgia, Grief: Emptiness; Pessimism: Disappointment, Discouragement, Despair
Mad: Anger, Hatred, Rage: Blame: Revenge, Spitefulness: Jealousy, Envy
Afraid: Fear, Anxiety, Doubt, Worry; Insecurity, Dread, Panic, Apprehensiveness; Confusion, Powerlessness Overwhelm, Bewilderment; Shame, Unworthiness; Guilt

(Note: If you feel "nothing", that is most likely a hidden emotion, i.e., a lack of feeling that results from overwhelming sadness, anger or fear. However, if you keep checking in, you'll be able to follow that numbness to its root, so you can surface your underlying emotions and increase your EQ.)

After you've done the check-in for a while, you can determine the top three emotions you experience regularly. These most significantly influence your Balancing Act and set your *emotional balance point*, i.e., the emotional state you live in most of the time. *Go to Section II to learn more (p 245).*

Chapter Five:

Build Healthier Habits

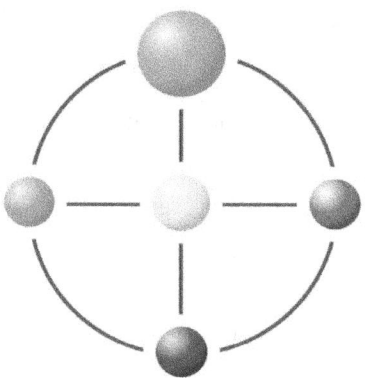

The techniques in this chapter will reduce stress so you: develop solid, more functional new habits; become more practical and realistic; generate and manage all the physical resources you need (including money, equipment, space and possessions); learn new ways to improve your health; feel secure, safe, stable; get much better organized; and become more dependable, with stronger follow-through.

Structure is the fifth Element of Success. In *The Balancing Act,* Structure corresponds to the direction of North (see image above), the classical element of Earth, and the Body. This fifth element is alive, like the Earth itself. Indeed, when Structure is aligned with the other Elements of Success, it becomes more like a solid-but-growing tree and much less like rigid concrete.

Because Structure is the most visible of all the Elements of Success, sometimes people try to resolve their problems by addressing this element first—or exclusively. Often however, the "root cause" of problems that eventually blossom in the Earth element actually lie deep below the surface, in other Elements of Success. It is also good to remember that you will only be able to adapt successfully within a changing environment if Structure is supported by all the other elements.

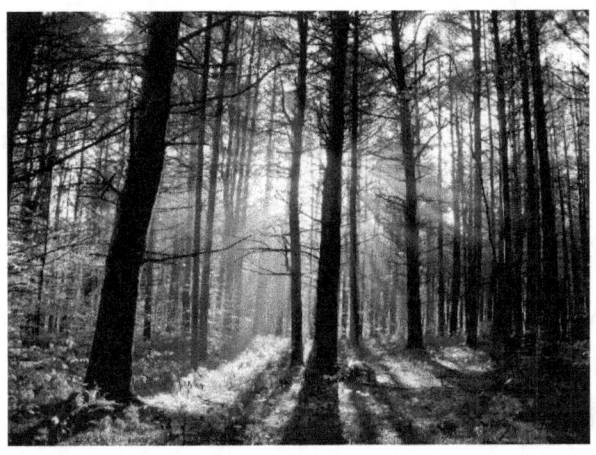

Structure helps you manage the resources you need to maintain your life. This element includes all the *infrastructure* (physical scaffolding) of your life, including: daily habits; living and working spaces; and the tools/resources you need to succeed (data, supplies, updated equipment—and of course, money). And if money issues are a major cause of your stress, know that you are not alone. According to a recent survey by the American Psychological Association, a full 75% of Americans list money as their primary stressor! Happily, you can find SOS relief for money stress not only in this chapter, but also in prior chapters (which will help you find and cure common root causes).

The element of Structure also includes the tangible outcomes of your efforts, i.e., the products and services you deliver to others—and for which they pay you. Structure is the steady, practical element that urges you to do today's work today, not hurry, and keep moving forward one step at a time so you can implement your strategy in an efficient way. Structure is careful and pragmatic; it seeks feedback from the environment so you can make necessary course corrections that keep you on track to your goals. In this way, Structure transforms you into a wise craftsman who measures twice and cuts once.

The fifth element helps you create a solid new structure that best suits your new life and work. Although you may hate doing so, growth requires you to break out of your comfort zone and let go of old habits and/or familiar structures. For example, if you've been pushing yourself at work, you may now notice new aches that demand you get up earlier so you can stretch before starting your day. If you enact this new habit, you're using Structure not only to feel better physically, but also to improve your attitude and energy.

This final element is where the rubber meets the road. Rather than allowing distress to weaken or rigidify your life-enhancing Structure, you can use the SOS techniques in this chapter to continue your upward Spiral of Success: i.e., first stopping to Reset from the Core, then directing your Mind to Reframe the situation, then having your Will manage your actions according to your new priorities, and next, allowing your Emotional GPS to guide you—all of which will show you how to build the best Structures to fit your new life. As the fifth step in the powerful TBA Change process, Structure requires you to "Repeat" new habits until you have implemented them as an integral part of your new, significantly improved daily reality. *For more information on Structure, read pages 165-176 in The Balancing Act.* (To read more about TBA or to purchase it, go to http://balance.thecoreporation.com.)

SOS Techniques that Build Healthier Habits:

69. Experience the Steadying Element of Structure (p 132)

70. Show Me the Money (p 132)

71. Hydrate Your Body (p 134)

72. Bless What You Eat and Drink (p 134)

73. Ear Massage (p 136)

74. Red Flag! (p 136)

75. S-t-r-e-t-c-h (p 138)

76. Brain Gym (p 141)

77. An Eat an Apple a Day (p 142)

78. Tea Time (p 142)

79. Remind Yourself to Eat Slowly (p 143)

80. You Snooze →You Win! (p 145)

81. Treat One of Your 5 Senses (p 145)

82. Take a Nature Break (p 147)

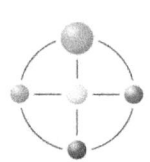

#69: Experience the Steadying Element of Structure

(4 minutes)

How to do SOS #69: Go to thecoreporation.com home page (or the sos_links page) and click on the Structure meditation audio. Then sit back, listen to my voice, and let me do all the work. *Go to Section II to learn more (p 246).*

#70: Show Me the Money

(4-6 minutes)

How to do SOS #70: In a now-classic movie scene, an athlete played by Cuba Gooding, Jr. demands that his sports agent, Jerry Maguire (played by Tom Cruise) "show me the money." Since money is a major stressor for most people, I'd like to show how you can take just a few moments to enliven this often-troubling aspect of the Earth element and break the death-grip it may have on your psyche.

You have SO many options here: You can "show me the money" by working directly with one of the SOS techniques in this chapter. Or, you may benefit from stepping back to reframe your thinking on the subject, then selecting another element to get to the root cause of your money problems (e.g., emotions, motivation, mental scripts/perceptions, and Core self-esteem).

Below I've listed just a few of the ways you can leverage any one of the Elements of Success to enliven, invigorate, and quickly improve your financial situation:

1. Use a Core breath technique to Reset, calm down, and regain esteem. (Try SOS #4 if you're super stressed.)

2. Reframe your money beliefs/perceptions and turn money stress into a teacher (SOS #31).

3. Activate your energy to launch a new money habit, make a sales call, or send an invoice (SOS #39).

4. Release hidden emotional scripts that block your monetary success (SOS #53 and SOS #54).

5. Take a small Structure step to implement an efficient money habit (e.g., input receipts into QuickBooks).

6. Remember "This too will Pass" (SOS #99); listen to Esther Hicks audio combining binaural beats with 3/5 stealth breath and "All is Well" money message (v=BBe1mfsbeWc).

Go to Section II to learn more (p 247).

#71: Hydrate Your Body

(1 minute)

How to do SOS #71: We don't need to belabor this point. You know you need to drink water. But this fact needs more emphasis when it comes to reducing your stress. Here's why:

One of the ways distress adversely affects your body is to cause dehydration. Ironically, not only does toxic stress cause dehydration, but also the reverse is true, i.e., dehydration creates more stress. After oxygen, water is the element most necessary to sustain human life. Insufficient water increases the stress hormone cortisol, which in turn results in all kinds of physical ills. Interestingly, dehydration mimics many other stress symptoms (increased heart rate, fatigue, hunger, headache, nausea), and it certainly can make any stress you're already feeling that much worse.

To make this simple practice more likely to happen—i.e., to invoke the 20-second rule (SOS #39), I suggest you keep a jug of water in your refrigerator or take a refillable (not throwaway) bottle wherever you go. *Go to Section II to learn more (p 249).*

#72: Bless What You Eat and Drink

(1 minute)

How to do SOS #72: Blessing what you eat and drink rather than mindlessly consuming these gifts is a great way to reduce your stress and improve your health. You have a thousand options to choose from here.

You can simply pause and breathe a few times before picking up your fork. You can say a few words that come naturally from your heart. You can silently thank the chain of people who brought this food and drink to your table: those who planted the seed, harvested the crop, took it to market, sold it to your family, and also those who cooked it and served it to you.

You could start with a childhood tradition or explore traditions from around the world that are intended to connect people to the Source that provides everything we eat and drink. And if meat is on the menu, you can borrow the Native American tradition of thanking the animal that gave its life for you. Our ancestors from all corners of the globe have recited these kinds of blessings for millennia. As it says in Exodus 23:25: "Worship the LORD your God, and his blessing will be on your food and water. I will take away sickness from among you."

If all the above is not reason enough for you to bless your food, just remember that unconscious eating and drinking adds pounds to your body and results in digestive and other illnesses. Eating too fast also winds up costing you more money because your body needs about 15-20 minutes to process the signals that you are full. (See SOS #79.)

So take action: turn off that TV, put down that book, walk away from your desk and find a pleasant spot for lunch, get out of email, turn off your phone, and close the lid on your laptop. Take a moment of "unplugged" time to relax in silence.

Then bless your food and drink and as promised, it will take sickness from you. *Go to Section II to learn more (p 249).*

#73: Ear Massage

(1-2 minutes)

How to do SOS #73: Apply light pressure to your earlobes, using your thumb and index finger. There are many ways to do ear massage; this version is called "ear rolling". Start at the top of your ear, where it meets your face. Move slowly up the outer rim of the ear to the top of your ear. The massaging motion is to very gently "unroll" or straighten the folds of the ears. Add a slow breath to this process to increase its SOS power.

Work your way along the path of the outer ear, moving down to the lobes at the bottom. You can do one round of ear massage in a minute or less. (But it feels so good you may find yourself wanting to do it again.) *Go to Section II to learn more (p 251).*

#74: Red Flag!

(2-4 minutes)

How to do SOS #74: Your body does a great job of sending "red flag" SOS signals. Although mental and emotional cues tend to surface before physical ones, many people are not aware of them. However, they may more readily notice the physical signs of a meltdown. All this SOS activity requires is for you to: a) observe/listen to your body's Red Flag signals so you can b) stop the downward spiral and c) act to reverse this toxic stress process before it gets worse.

For example, let's say that your typical early warning signal for the emotion of anger is feeling as if your gut is twisting into a knot. Whenever you recognize that physical cue, you will have a real chance to stop yourself before you say something hurtful to another person or erupt into violence (both of which will only make matters much worse). Interrupting a meltdown could involve any one of the SOS techniques you've found effective: for example doing the ER breath, commanding yourself to "Stop it!", taking a walk outdoors to calm down, or doing emotional release techniques (such as EFT or PSTEC).

It is important to take strong and immediate action to interrupt this downward spiral because if ignore such red flag signals, you will add a whole other set of problems, new drama, and even more stress to your current crisis.

This SOS technique is also good to use when you see a loved one breaking down; noticing red flag signals could allow you to help them &/or keep yourself out of danger. For example, you can teach children to watch for physical signals that alert them to move away from a bully's reach (or keep them from bullying others). You can help a friend short-circuit an ill-advised action, stay out of your boss' way when no good will come of a conversation, or remove yourself from the danger of abuse.

All you have to do for this SOS activity is observe how YOUR body talks to you when it's stressed (everyone is different). Common physical warning signs include: jitters/twitching; grinding teeth; tightening face; getting a cold or becoming ill; stuttering/becoming speechless; balling hands into fists; eyes feeling sore or tears starting; ears getting red; face contorting; chest or back pains; shortage of breath, dry mouth; upset stomach; tense muscles; overeating comfort food; nightmares; sleep deprivation; memory loss and inability to concentrate. (Interestingly, some people say that they literally "see red" before turning from nice Dr. Jekyll into homicidal Mr. Hyde.) *Go to Section II to learn more (p 251).*

#75: S-t-r-e-t-c-h

(4-6 minutes)

How to do SOS #75: Stretching feels good: it releases physical kinks, increases overall strength, improves posture, boosts self-esteem—and increases your attractiveness! (You look better after stretching because you are more relaxed and the blood flow has improved throughout your whole body.) And when you add slow breathing to stretching, it multiplies the positive health effects and makes stretching much easier. (I also recommend "mini-stretching"—just a few seconds of movement whenever it occurs to you will add up to big benefits over time.)

Another benefit of gently stretching your muscles is that it reduces the likelihood of injury from more intense exercising—which is why stretching is used by serious athletes to warm up before, and cool down after, their workouts.

If you've already tried stretching or yoga, you know how wonderful it can feel. There are hundreds of ways to do stretching. There's even a whole school of sitting-at-your-desk yoga poses, so you have no excuse whatsoever to miss the advantages of this rich tradition. If you're new to stretching, I suggest the following simple exercise to start:

1. Stand tall with your feet together, shoulders relaxed, weight evenly distributed through your soles, arms at your sides.

2. Take a deep breath. Raise both hands overhead, palms facing, with your arms straight. Reach up toward the sky with your fingertips.

3. Continue breathing deeply while you hold this pose. Do a body scan to loosen any muscles that are tense. Continue steady breathing so muscles can stretch a bit higher.

4. Then, on a slow exhalation, bring your palms down until they are in front of your chest. Release the pose and allow your arms to return to the sides of your body.

5. Relax. Breathe in and out as you feel the benefits of this stretch. Repeat this pose as often as you wish.

Sun Salutation: This combination of yogic moves is one of my all-time favorite stretching activities. After you've mastered a few beginning stretches, you may want to try this out. The Sun Salutation is a designed to wake you up, work the whole body, benefit all your internal organs, and rejuvenate your energy. Once you've learned the solar salutation, you can do a full whole round in 2-3 minutes—so it's easy to do two or three full rounds within 6 minutes.

You can learn how to do this series of moves by reading this illustrated article (sharecare.com/health/fitness-exercise/article/yoga-sun-salutation) or by following either of these videos:

- Instructions #1 (4 minutes; v=yuvfHTaftLQ)
- Instructions #2 (7 minutes; v=yuvfHTaftLQ).

Slanting: And finally, a passive form of stretching—where you let gravity do all the work for you—is "slanting" or "inversion". You can try this technique by using a well-padded ironing board or by putting cushions on a wood plank. If you like it, get yourself a slant board. All you need to do is: lie on the board with your feet at the top of a slight incline. The degree of inversion depends on your preferences; start with a 6" incline and see how that feels. Slanting has many health benefits, so it's worth your time to try it out. (Caveat: If you have any of the following health problems, DO NOT do slanting: high blood pressure, hemorrhages, retinal detachment, tuberculosis, strokes, ulcers, appendicitis, or if you're pregnant.) *Go to Section II to learn more (p 252).*

#76: Brain Gym

(4-6 minutes)

How to do SOS #76: A great way to relieve stress, get unstuck and increase energy is to do some brain gym exercises. Although brain gym was designed for children, I find them useful for all ages. (Myself included.)

The point in all brain gym exercises is to have your limbs cross your body's midline. My favorite one is the cross-crawl. Here's how to do it: Stand up, and then begin marching in place, swinging your arms as if you were in a parade. (C'mon, loosen up!) Next, lift your ankle in front of you and tap it with the *opposite side* hand. Depending on your flexibility, you could touch your elbow to your opposite knee. (Caution: Start slow and easy, especially if you're stiff.) Repeat this as many times as you need, until your body feels much better and you've shaken out all those kinks.

Clearly you'll have to adjourn to some quiet space to do brain gym exercises (unless you have your own office or some really fun colleagues who will join you, rather than rain on your parade). There are also some brain gym exercises you can do while sitting; these can be useful when you're stuck in traffic.

And, if it's your children who are stressed—or who are causing you stress, don't hesitate to make this a family event. Put on some music and enjoy this activity together. You'll be doing your children, yourself, your spouse, and all their teachers and friends a great favor. *Go to Section II to learn more (p 254).*

#77: Eat an Apple a Day

(2-3 minutes)

How to do SOS #77: The old adage "An apple a day keeps the doctor away" has a scientific basis: apples are a rich source of potassium, antioxidants, and vitamins B6 and C. What's more, they are a naturally sweet alternative to more sugary snacks.

I actually do eat an apple a day! Indeed, I find that eating half of a sweet apple an hour or so before bedtime helps me sleep better. Since I have as many worries as the next person that can keep me tossing and turning rather than happily drifting off, I have tested many research based sleep-enhancing techniques on myself, and then have adopted a few that work well for me. Eating an apple before bedtime is the most natural, simple and sustainable sleep-enhancing technique I know.

Go to Section II to learn more (p 255).

#78: Tea Time

(6 minutes)

How to do SOS #78: If you've been working at your desk for a long time, take a break and get yourself a cup of tea to refresh and restart yourself. (Often people take longer tea breaks, but you can get significant stress relief in just a few minutes by making some fresh tea and bringing it back to your desk.)

Breaking for tea is a time honored stress-relieving tradition that is used around the globe. In fact, teatime is so important that labor strikes have resulted in factories when managers tried to cut out their workers tea breaks. And, have you ever noticed that pretty much every British film has a moment when one of the central characters tries to ease someone's distress with an across-the-society question that goes something like this: "Would you like a cuppa tea, dearie?" or "Charles, please tell the maid to bring some tea for our guests."

In America and much of the modern world, teatime has been replaced by coffee breaks, which serve much the same de-stressing function. *Go to Section II to learn more (p 255).*

#79: Remind Yourself to Eat Slowly

(1-2 minutes)

How to do SOS #79: Mom was right! If you remind yourself to slow down while eating, you'll gain many health benefits. Hopefully you have just blessed your food and drink (SOS #72), so this stress-reduction process follows naturally. All you have to do before picking up your fork, spoon, or chopsticks, is to take a breath and remind yourself to eat slowly while you take the time to completely chew your food. If you notice yourself mindlessly or rapidly munching, stop. Put down your eating utensil, breathe, remind yourself again to eat slowly— then start over. (Your Mom will be proud.)

There are all kinds of benefits from eating slowly: your brain has time to realize you're full, so you'll consume fewer calories. This translates not only to reduced stress but also to weight control, money savings, improved digestion and better health.

Truth be told, most of us treat our meals like "fast food" even when they're nothing of the sort. Fortunately, we can unlearn the dysfunctional behavior of eating too fast. Here are some tips for succeeding with this new habit. Start by experimenting with just ONE of the below tips to replace your current eating habits. Then over time move on to integrate other tips until you have completely changed your way of eating:

- Sit down to eat (but not at your desk!)

- Savor your food. Really taste it.

- Chew your food thoroughly rather than gulping it down.

- Put down your fork, pause and breathe between bites.

- Take smaller bites.

- Focus on what you're doing; don't let your mind wander.

- Turn off the TV or computer so you are less distracted.

- Stay mindful of what you're eating.

- Put on music that slows you down.

- Make meals social occasions; talk with people you love.

Go to Section II to learn more (p 256).

#80: You Snooze →You Win!

(5-6 minute)

How to do SOS #80: Just close your eyes and relax. Find a quiet place to take a power nap. Set an alarm for the time you have available for the nap. Your body restores whenever you unplug, whether it's a super-short catnap, a siesta, or a great night sleep. (I like to supplement my catnaps with meditation music to help me relax more deeply in whatever time I have.)

It is no accident that siestas are used the whole world over to reset, recalibrate, and refresh. In fat, napping is a normal part of daily sleep patterns for about *one-third* of people in the world. In sharp contrast, Americans are among the most sleep-deprived people in the world—and other industrialized countries seem to be doing their best to "catch-up". So, if you're feeling sluggish during the day, you might try a little snooze rather than reach for another cup of coffee or a sugary/fatty snack. *Go to Section II to learn more (p 257).*

#81: Treat One of Your 5 Senses

(4-6 minutes)

How to do SOS #81: Take a break to indulge one of your five senses. This will help you enjoy the vitality of your body in the moment. Maybe your nerves are frayed from the corrosive sounds of street or workplace noise. Perhaps your eyes feel as if they're swelling shut or a headache is starting because you've been at the computer all day. Maybe you're eating too fast and not really tasting your food.

All you have to do for this practice is notice which one of your five senses is being over-used, and then reset your physical state by taking a few minutes to be kind to your body. This SOS tool is fast, direct, and very practical. Indeed, any of the below suggestions can turn into a instant sensory-focused meditation:

Hearing: You could turn on relaxing music, shut everything off to enjoy silence, or put on a sound cancelling noise machine. Then sit quietly and enjoy.

Taste: Remind yourself to thoroughly chew your food so you fully savor all the tastes. Choose tasty, nourishing food to eat.

Smell: Our ancient ancestors used their powerful sense of smell to avoid danger, and today we can use it to relieve stress. Research on Aromatherapy indicates that carefully chosen scents can eliminate pain and calm emotions. I recommend finding pure products at your local health food store, and suggest you start with lavender for relaxation.

Sight: Rub your hands together and rest them on your eyes and/or rest with your eyes closed for a few moments. You can gaze softly at a candle flame, some beautiful scenery, or watch the ocean's soothing waves to give your sense of sight a treat.

Touch: Skin is the largest organ in the body, and touch is the only way to nourish it. Make an appointment with a masseuse. Buy a couples massage book and set a date with your mate.

Give yourself an ear massage (see SOS #73) or find foot, hand, face massage instructions to try. Do some simple "spa" self-care: give yourself a manicure or pedicure; get your hair done, etc. Give someone a hug—which means YOU get one too. (See SOS #64.) *Go to Section II to learn more (p 258).*

#82: Take a Break in Nature

(6 minutes--or longer if you wish)

How to do SOS #82: Taking a break outdoors is an awesome de-stressing tool, largely because Nature does most of the work for you. It facilitates a sense of peace and relaxation by helping you connect at a visceral level with whatever you feel is at the source of all this beauty. Nature is also a great "midwife" for intuition (in a quiet natural setting, most people find it easier to hear their intuition talking to them).

All you have to do is unplug from "civilization" for a few moments. Turn off all your electronic devices and go to some quiet natural spot near you. Happily, even in a city there are many places where you can take a short outdoor break. For example, you can choose a park to have your lunch, take a short detour to or from work to walk through a tree-lined street, stop to admire a garden, or sit by a river for even a few moments. To get started with this activity, make a list of the parks, nature trails, hiking areas, or arboretums near your workplace or home. Locate a park just off your commute route. See where you can go fishing or rent kayaks for an outing this coming weekend. Listen to news and weather reports for notices of meteor showers or possible days off to play in the snow or dance in the rain.

When I worked in Boston's downtown financial district, I would sometimes take what I thought of as a "Nature detour"; i.e., between one meeting and the next, I'd find a bench on the harbor where I could bask in the sun for just a few moments, drink in the ocean air and watch the seagulls trail the fishing boats. It was lovely micro-vacation. And when I lived in the Midwest, nothing was more gratifying than walking in the woods, sitting lakeside, watching the changing weather roll by, or gazing up at a clear, star-studded night sky. (Heaven!)

You can take a Nature break by sitting in your backyard or a neighborhood park where you can feel grass under your feet, put your fingers in the soil, watch local fauna going about their business, lean against a tree, turn your face to drink in the sun's rays, feel the breeze on your closed eyes, watch clouds changing shapes, or listen to bird song. And, if you're indoors, just pause a moment to watch the beauty of the day parade past your window. *Go to Section II to learn more (p 258).*

#83: Schedule Stress Breaks

(1 minute)

How to do SOS #83: Turn your calendar from a stress-maker into a stress-reliever by scheduling *breaks* in it. I find that if I block out some SOS time in my calendar, it becomes "real" and the likelihood of my actually taking a time-out increases exponentially. (It is in my calendar; ergo, it exists.)

With this small action, you are making a promise to yourself. And, if you add a reminder alarm to that scheduled break, your odds of getting out of whatever rut you're in and taking a soul-nourishing break are further multiplied. What's more: you can use this tool to increase the possibility of doing *other* SOS activities. (Just note them in your schedule.)

The first step is simple and very quick: Put a time-stamped reminder down in black and white in your calendar. I find that making this appointment with myself elevates it to the same status as the meetings that occur before and after it.

If you wish, you can leave the nature of the break up to your whim of the moment, but I find I do better if I specify the nature of the break ("Take walk" or "Stop by library" or "Call sibs"). This helps me keep my priorities straight, and also reduces stress by reminding me of something enjoyable I can look forward to doing soon. *Go to Section II to learn more (p 259).*

#84: Get a Boost from Brain Food

(1-2 minutes)

How to do SOS #84: When choosing what to eat, you can decide to simultaneously nourish your body, decrease stress and eat smarter with many tasty "brain food" options. Here is a list of top brain-food choices that I have compiled from several sources: berries (especially blueberries), nuts (walnuts), seeds (pumpkin), avocados, olive oil, spinach, beets, garlic, tomatoes, sardines, oily fish (wild salmon), sage (how apt), black currants, and whole grains (wheat germ). And some researchers even included coffee and dark chocolate on their brain-food lists. (Thank you, kind researchers!)

In contrast, "dumbing-down" foods are high in processed sugars and readily available as fast foods. Added sugar (vs. naturally occurring sugar) adversely affects your brain, resulting in memory loss, learning disorders, mood swings, depression and possibly dementia. Most of us know that high-sugar foods are long-term stressors for our bodies, but now we're learning that they also have an adverse impact on brain functioning. (Who knew?) *Go to Section II to learn more (p 260).*

#85: Clean-Sort-Move-File

(5-6 minutes)

How to do SOS #85: All this SOS process requires is for you to spend a few minutes cleaning, sorting, filing, or moving things around so your work and living spaces become functional and beautiful.

Clutter, dust, dirt, and holding on to physical items that no longer fit your life, all create stress. When you can't find a file you need, you're likely to get agitated and lose time. When papers are in piles, you may be too embarrassed to bring guests or clients into the room. When you haven't removed dust or vacuumed the rugs, it's actually unhealthy. Opening your closet to see old clothes in styles and sizes that don't suit you is downright depressing. And, furniture that is largely unused only takes up valuable space.

Removing these eyesores is an SOS technique that can relax your whole body and make you feel better every time you walk into that room. Happily, all it takes is a few minutes at a time to put your house and life into better order.

I like to combine this activity with music and turn it into exercise. (See Short Bursts, SOS #42). It works really well to transform these often-avoided tasks into stress-busting activities. Plus, it's *amazing* how much headway you can make with these short bursts of cleaning, sorting, filing, and moving things (and yourself) around.

Go to Section II to learn more (p 260).

Chapter Six:

Experience Greater Ease

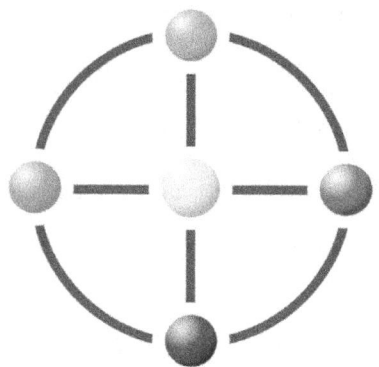

The techniques in this chapter will reduce stress so you: have a greater experience of ease, flow, and thriving; allow good luck and whatever you desire to be yours; become aware of all the infrastructures that surround and support you; and feel more deeply connected to, and gratitude for, the Context, Source, Whole that facilitates your individual life, work, relationships.

Synergy is the Context that connects all the Elements of Success. It corresponds to the strong interconnecting lines in the image above and, in classical thought, the directions of *Above* and *Below*. And in human beings, Synergy can be thought of as the creative, evolutionary force that lives inside us, surrounds us, and connects us to all that exists.

Synergy is another way of saying that the Whole is greater than the sum of its parts. It has been called *flow*, and the ancient alchemists referred to it as "the miracles of one thing".

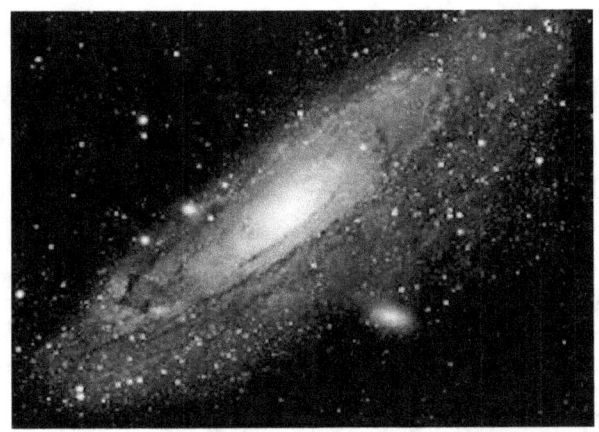

Synergy can help you connect-the-dots and align the five Elements of Success so you experience ease, thrive personally, allow good things to come into your life, and produce breakthrough results that seem miraculous. When all the elements are balanced and integrated, each one positively affects the others.

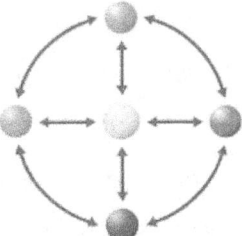

The resulting Synergy acts like a chemical formula: it sparks a virtuous chain reaction, initiates an upward spiral of growth, and generates positive ripple effects that multiply your efforts so you become "all that you can be" (and maybe even a bit more than you ever thought possible). Synergy produces an overflowing, evolutionary "excess of life" with which you can transcend prior limitations.

Another way to say this is that Synergy sparks a healing cycle that affects not only your life, but also positively influences many others with whom you interact…and perhaps even helps people you'll never know!

Hence the Native American belief that when you heal yourself, you heal seven generations backwards and forwards. My corollary is: when you heal yourself, you heal seven levels outward to family, friends, community and the world.

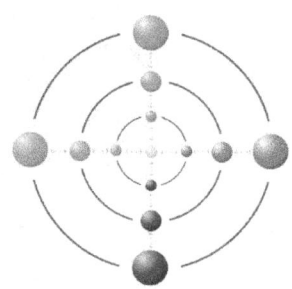

Unfortunately, distress occurs when the Elements of Success are not aligned. (And in turn, this toxic stress further weakens the links among the elements). Simply put, a lack of Synergy makes everything you do much harder. It may feel as if you can't catch a break; that the only luck you have is "bad" luck. Distress is also likely to result in feelings of isolation, a general sense of unhappiness, and the belief that you'll have to work very hard to get anything you want. However, you can use Synergy to turn stress into an ally who helps you find the root, underlying causes of your problems.

When Synergy provides a contextual, big-picture perspective, it starts working for you: things you hadn't noticed previously now grab your attention; people you've wanted to meet are suddenly shaking your hand at a networking event; friends make new suggestions that hadn't occurred to them previously; important calls come seemingly out of nowhere.

At first, this shift in your "luck" may take you by surprise. But don't fight it; experiencing Synergy means that you're on track and all the Elements of Success are working together for you. Your efforts will increasingly move under their own steam. What a relief! It will feel more as if you're watching a ball roll downhill versus having to push a boulder up a mountain.

You can use the SOS techniques in this chapter to leverage and enhance every step you've taken thus far in your evolutionary Spiral of Success. In the TBA Change model, Synergy is the final step in which you connect, align and balance all the Elements of Success. In so doing, you can fully *reclaim* all your power and create a *miracle* in your life. (Note that *reclaim* and *miracle* are anagrams.) *For more information on Synergy, read pages 215-226 in The Balancing Act* (To read more about TBA or to purchase it, go to http://balance.thecoreporation.com.)

SOS Techniques to help you Experience Greater Ease:

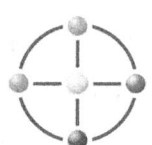

#86: Experience the Flow of Synergy

(3-4 minutes)

<u>How to do SOS #86:</u> Go to thecoreporation.com home page (or the sos_links page) and click on the Synergy meditation audio. Then sit back, listen to my voice, and let me do all the work. *Go to Section II to learn more (p 261).*

#87: Ho'oponopono

(6 - 60 seconds)

<u>How to do SOS #87:</u> All you have to do for this SOS technique is silently repeat this four-part phrase to yourself:

I'm sorry. Please forgive me. Thank you. I love you.

That's it! (For extra benefit, breathe slowly.) And, feel free to repeat it as frequently as you wish, whenever it occurs to you.

This blessing comes from *Ho'oponopono*, a compassionate healing technique based on ancient Hawaiian shamanism—which holds that we are all connected to each other through invisible threads (a bit like super-string theory in physics). Therefore, when a problem affects one of us, it affects all of us. Similarly, each one of us shares, very subtly, in both the cause and the cure of the problem.

I find that this simple phrase provides immediate relief when I experience something that disturbs me—an annoying or aggressive person, a disturbing news story. I find it particularly helpful when I feel out-of-sorts, confounded by a serious problem, or powerlessness about disasters a world away because it allows me to transform any stress I'm feeling into an opportunity for connection, forgiveness and healing.

(Note: I do an even shorter version when nothing is troubling me and I am spilling over with good feelings, i.e., "Thank you. I love you." I especially enjoy this when walking outdoors.)

Here's another variation on the Ho'oponopono theme of "forgive and be forgiven":

1. Bring to mind someone about whom you have negative feelings (start with small irritations and work your way up to real grievances once you've gotten the hang of this).

2. See that person clearly in your mind, standing a few feet in front of you.

3. Ask that person to forgive you for anything you've done to harm him or her. (Pause.) Imagine that person's forgiveness being sent to you. Allow it to settle inside you; say thank you.

4. Then send your forgiveness to that person for any harm you experienced. (Pause.) Realize that, by forgiving, you release this negativity and open a space where ease and peace can take its place. (Pause.) Done.

Go to Section II to learn more (p 262).

#88: The Healing Code

(6 minutes)

How to do SOS #88: This powerful self-help technique, created by Alexander Lloyd in 2001, is as easy as A-B-C!

A. Identify emotional roots: When you experience distress or pain, identify how you feel about it (for example, anger, fear, sadness). If possible, call to mind a time when you experienced this kind of pain or difficult emotion. (For example, I fell on the ice when I was twelve, bruised my tailbone, and was in great pain for days. I was angry for having fallen and I was also afraid I'd never get better). Then rate these old emotions from 1-10, with 10 being the most severe.

B. Set your intention: Tailor the following statement to your situation: "I pray that all known and hidden negative images, unhealthy beliefs, destructive cellular memories, and all resulting physical issues *(this back pain)* related to the feelings of *(anger and fear)* be found, opened and healed by filling me with the love, light and life of God. I also pray that the effectiveness of this healing be increased 100 times or more."

C. Do the Code: Point your ten fingers at four spots on your head for 30 seconds each. These are:

> 1. The bridge between your eyebrows;
>
> 2. In front of your throat's Adam's apple;
>
> 3. Both sides of your jaw; and
>
> 4. Both sides of your temple.

Hold your fingers about 2-3 inches from your head, imagining that the fingertips are like flashlights sending energy to these spots. Do three rounds of 2 minutes each. While doing the Healing Code process, replace the distressing emotion by focusing on feeling a positive emotion, &/or smiling, &/or repeating a prayer, a meaningful phase or one of Lloyd's "truth focus" statements.

Optional: Before starting, rate the strength of your current pain or stress from 1-10. Then when done, rate it again to see how much it has changed. You can also check back on the originating emotion to see if that older memory has eased at all.

Go to Section II to learn more (p 263).

#89: Express Gratitude

(4-6 minutes)

How to do SOS #89: Feeling and expressing gratitude is one of the fastest routes to releasing toxic stress. When you're upset by something that's going wrong, stop. Then take a time out to count your blessings. (I mean that literally – count them!)

Just grab a notepad and do a brain-dump of everything that is going right for you. Write whatever pops into your mind. When done, reread your list and put your current problem into this context. You will notice that the problem seems to have shrunk in relative size, loosened its grip on you, and is not nearly the catastrophe you thought only a few minutes ago.

I've been doing variations of this exercise for many years, and have to say that I always feel better when I'm doing a gratitude practice regularly. I keep a small journal and write down, first thing in the morning, just *3 things from the past 24 hours* for which I'm particularly grateful. (Usually I wind up with more.) I also have found that remembering good things from the day is a terrific way to slide effortlessly into a good night's sleep.

Amazingly, researchers in positive psychology discovered that gratitude has a long-lasting impact on happiness. Subjects who did this daily "3 things" gratitude practice not only reported being significantly happier than a control group at the time— they *remained significantly happier for 6 months* after the study.

Variations of this practice include completing the sentence "I am so grateful and happy that _____". Or, you can be really bold, push back on the static concept of time, and assume that whatever you strongly desire is already on its way to you: "I am so grateful and happy now that _____ (this good thing) has happened".

You can also do gratitude practices with loved ones (e.g., do an out-loud gratitude practice with your children at the dinner table or bedtime to help them remember and relive the good things they experienced that day.) Or, you can say thank you to someone who deserves appreciation (SOS #65). And, last but not least, you can do one of my favorite activities: while walking, silently say "thank you" to express your joy, love and gratitude for the myriad forms of beauty all around you.

My clients who embrace some form of gratitude practice are the ones who move most quickly to new lives of their own making. So, if you want to become more immune to stress and more likely to succeed—just weave gratitude into the fabric of your daily life. *Go to Section II to learn more (p 265).*

#90: OM Sounding

(4-6 minutes)

How to do SOS #90: "OM" is considered by many traditions to be the seed-sound that created the universe and that contains all the elements inside it. It feels SO good when you do it. You can simply listen to (or sound along with) the below audios. Obviously, if other people are near you at work or home, just listen—you don't want to annoy them. However, you will get the most benefit from this technique if you do it out loud so the OM sound vibrates fully throughout your body. Notice that "Om" ("Aum") is formed by three distinct sounds: "Ah –ooo –mmm."

#1 Om Sounding. (v=0PJx8PE_GVM; 6 minutes)

#2. Om Sounding. (v=yoYrLM5rGX8; extended)

Practitioners of OM sounding suggest that you inhale deeply, and then on one continual out-breath intone: "Ahh" (3 seconds) – "oooo" (5 seconds) – "mmmmm" (6 seconds or longer). Just do a guesstimate; don't use a stopwatch. It's much easier to get a feel for the relative timing by doing a finger count to make sure each successive part of the AUM is slightly longer than the one before. Once you've done this a few times, you can drop the count and settle into simply experiencing the beauty of the sound. *Go to Section II to learn more (p 266).*

#91: I Am That I Am

(6 seconds)

How to do SOS #91: This technique is so ancient that it's difficult to determine where and with whom it originated. ("I AM" is a variation of "OM" or "AUM".)

I learned this technique as a sitting meditation, but I love to do it while walking outside, in time with my breath and steps—all while observing the beauty of the environment surrounding me. The way I do this is to silently repeat this phrase on both the in-breath and out breath.

Doing this phrase very slowly with deep breathing stretches it to six seconds—so feel free to repeat it as often as you wish. *Go to Section II to learn more (p 268).*

#92: When in Doubt, Pray

(1 minute or as long as you desire)

How to do SOS #92: We often pray during times when we are the most distressed. (Even people with little faith can return to the comfort of prayer during crises). No matter what your belief system, you can dialogue internally with God, a higher Power, or appeal to the scientific forces and/or organizing intelligence that propels the Universe. In our darkest hours, sometimes prayer provides a powerful Context of greater meaning that helps us more wisely navigate our difficulties.

I believe that the best prayers are not necessarily those we memorized in childhood, but rather those that leap naturally from our hearts to meet the situation with which we are struggling. There are countless ways to pray. For example, we may suddenly hear ourselves begging God for a big favor. Or, we may prefer prayers that focus on thanking, connecting, dialoguing, listening, and coming to a sense of peace.

If you find yourself at a loss for words, I have listed some beautiful prayers from around the world in Learn More. And, a final word about this activity: adding your breath to your prayers will help you slow down, settle down, and bring your full heart and mind into the prayer. *Go to Section II to learn more (p 268).*

#93: All is Well

(30 -60 seconds)

How to do SOS #93: When you're losing your perspective or becoming overwhelmed by excessive stress, try this affirmation to help you put your difficulties into a larger context. It will reduce your resistance, stop you from creating catastrophes, and allow some space for good things to happen instead.

I think of this simple phrase as a blessing not only for myself, but also for everything and everything around me. I came across this affirmative prayer when I studied the life and music of St. Hildegard of Bingen, a 12th century mystic and holistic healer. She is reported to have stated:

> *All shall be well, All shall be well,*
>
> *and all manner of thing shall be well.*

The present-day holistic healer Louise Hays has her own version of this timeless affirmation:

> *All is well. Everything is working out for my highest good.*
>
> *Out of this situation only good will come. I am safe.*

I find that by saying either one of these phrases, I can quickly calm myself down. See if you find it as comforting as countless others have. And lastly, I recommend this well-being meditation by Ester Hicks that sets the 3/5 breath-count to music (v=-waD9FhOk98). *Go to Section II to learn more (p 271).*

#94: Healing Circle

(5-6 minutes)

How to do SOS #94: *SOS: Switch Off Stress* is based on *The Balancing Act* and it, in turn is based on the global archetypal template of the center and four directions. When these five elements (which represent your Soul, Mind, Will, Emotions, Body) are aligned, the result is Synergy, balance, and wellbeing. You can make up your own version of a healing circle to help you de-stress, put everything in perspective, and call up your power. Here is an example of a Healing Circle that borrows from the traditions of indigenous North Americans. You can do this process in your imagination or move physically through the following steps.

1. Center. Wherever you stand is the Center of the Wheel. Remind yourself of your calm Core and feel the "essential" energy that is the best part of you. (Your Soul.)

2. East. Turn, bow, and take a few steps toward the East, in the direction of your right hand. Remind yourself of how the classical element of Air (your Mind) can make you feel uplifted and optimistic. Pause. Move back to the center.

3. *South.* Next turn toward, bow, and take a few steps behind you to the South. Remind yourself of the powerful energy of Fire and feel that burning energy inside you. (This corresponds to your Will.) Pause. Move back to the Center.

4. *West.* Now move a few steps to the West, and remind yourself of the flow of Water so that you acknowledge and strengthen your love for others. (This corresponds to your Emotions.) Pause. Go back to the Center.

5. *North.* Now move to the North, and call to mind the solid strength of the Earth element that keeps you grounded so you can stay practical and realistic. (This element corresponds to your Body.) Pause. Move back to Center.

6. *Above and Below.* While standing in the Center, think about the powerful Context that holds you. Call upon the sacred space that surrounds you. (Above and Below.) Pause. End.

Go to Section II to learn more (p 271).

#95: The 5 Element Mantra

(6 seconds to as long as you wish)

How to do SOS #95: Another way to cast a healing circle to manage your stress is by repeating this powerful phrase. All the classical Elements of Success are contained in this ancient invocation that is used widely in India and other Far East countries. In fact, this 5-element mantra is considered sacred by the tradition of Shaivism, a form of Hinduism.

The sacred phrase is: "Om Namah Shivaya". In this mantra <u>Na</u> is Earth, <u>Ma</u> is Water, <u>Śi</u> is Fire, <u>Vā</u> is Air, and <u>Ya</u> is Essence. <u>Om</u> or Aum is believed to be the originating "seed sound" that created the universe and contains all of these elements.

This phase can be repeated silently or out loud; it can also be sung. Adding the breath is part of the meditative practice. As you repeat this phrase, think of these sounds aligning, balancing, and healing every aspect of you: your Soul, Mind, Will, Emotions, Body—and even rippling out to positively affect the world that holds you. *Go to Section II to learn more (p 272).*

#96: Find the Roots of Your Distress

(2-4 minutes)

How to do SOS #96: There are a number of ways to discover the roots of your distress and prevent the repetition of the same or similar problems. All you need to do is ask questions regarding how this problem came to be, and then pause to contemplate the answers. Often the toxic stress you feel is a symptom of chronic, underlying, more serious problems. These latter are the "root causes" to which I refer. So, when you next feel overly stressed, become a detective to see if you can follow your distress all the way back to the scene of the crime.

Hopefully the answers to the below questions will help you understand what's going on, and maybe even point out how you can correct the problem at its roots. Make notes of any answers you find. Examples of this inquiry process include:

Option One:

Asking open-ended questions that begin with: "What...? Where...? Why...? When...? How...? Who...?" For example, "Where did this problem first surface?" "Why does it bother me so much?" "Who contributed to it &/or who can help fix it?" Etc.

Option Two:

Asking the question "Why...?" 5 times. That is, ask and get an answer to the first "Why...?" Then that answer is likely to suggest another "why" question that takes you deeper. And so on. For example, Question #1: "Why don't I spend more time with my friends?" Answer #1: "Because I'm too tired after work." Q2: "Why am I so tired after work?" A2: "I spend 12 hours a day working plus an hour commuting each way—of course I'm tired!" Q #3: "Why do I have 14 hour work days?" Etc.

Option Three:

Asking a series of questions like those below to discover the roots of potentially toxic stress.

A. When did this distress begin (or when did I first notice it)?

B. What was the first symptom I noticed?

C. What happened before; i.e., what set off the chain-reaction?

D. When have prior (similar) problems happened?

E. Is there a pattern to how & when this problem occurs?

Go to Section II to learn more (p 272).

#97: Get the Binaural Beat

(6 minutes or longer if you choose)

How to do SOS #97: Binaural audios are a "short-cut" relaxation tool for all the too-stressed-to-take-time-out-to-mediate people, making it a great SOS technique. This exciting "whole brain" process represents a wonderful intersection between ancient meditation techniques, brain research, and modern technology. Binaural audios are developed with *multivariate resonance technology*, which gently eases people into a natural meditative state.

The sensation of auditory binaural beats occurs when two sounds of nearly similar frequencies are played, one to each ear with stereo headphones. The brain integrates the two signals, producing a sensation of a *third sound* called the binaural beat; this process relaxes the whole brain.

This first binaural sample is called Balance (v=By__pQ8ju0w)—and it will certainly help you regain your balance when you're feeling stressed. It's from the good people at Mind Valley, who have researched and developed many OmHarmonics sound tracks that allow you to enter an almost instant state of meditation. You can listen for just 6 minutes, or longer if you choose. Always use headsets with these audios to get the most benefit. (This link has a 1½-minute introduction by MindValley's CEO). Or you can enjoy a video set to the same track (v=qSEyKMApVAs&list=PL5MudRtHvQANpXEYTY0QrRN0MM hJaBD5n). *Go to Section II to learn more (p 273).*

#98: Portable Spa Treatment

(6 minutes)

How to do SOS #98: You can use this 5 Elements Portable Spa treatment to relax anytime, anywhere. Just follow these steps:

Step 1. Go to the Portable Spa Center. Start by sitting comfortably in your chair, hands resting in your lap. You may want to close your eyes to shut out any stimuli around you. Begin by taking a deep breath in, then a long breath out. After a few deep breaths, move to a simple Core Breath technique. (For example, "Breathe in – 2 – 3; breathe out – 2 – 3 – 4 – 5.)." Continue this process until your muscles relax, your mind becomes calm and steady, and your stress melts away.

Step 2. What's on My Mind? While continuing your breath count, notice what's on your mind. What thoughts pop up, trying to get your attention? Simply notice them, thank them, and write them down so you can deal with them later. (This keeps you Mind from unproductive looping that would spoil your whole spa experience.) Now return to your Portable Spa Center and relax, knowing you will be able to take better care of problems later because you took this restorative time-out.

Step 3. Commit to Action. From the list you made in step 2, highlight any particularly stressful items. Beside those items, note some possible actions you could take to make changes that will reduce your overall stress.

From the many things your Mind says need tending to: decide what is in your power to change. Commit to taking ONE action. After you're done with the spa, you can determine details about how to achieve that goal within a specified timeline.

Step 4. The Warm Smile. Now that your mind is emptying, you can really relax. You're committed to taking action. Stress can stop punishing you for ignoring it. Return to your breath count. You will need both internal and external support to help you accomplish your goal. Internal emotional support comes from knowing that you're on your way to success. Bask in the warm glow of that realization by allowing a slow, warm smile to light up your face. Now *feel* this smile flow through your whole body like a smooth, healing potion that sends a signal to change your body chemistry, upping your odds of success.

Step 5. Make Room for a New Habit. And lastly, it's time to think about what resources, structures, &/or new habits you need to implement to achieve your goal. Write down some options for you to do immediately. Once started with this pragmatic, real-life experiment, you can make course corrections as required. When you leave the spa, you'll have a chance to start by changing one small new habit—but this time, you'll have all the Elements of Success backing you up!

Step 6. Watch for Synergy. As you leave the spa, allow yourself to thoroughly enjoy how great you feel, from head to toe. Let yourself fully experience any good luck that happens as you move through the day, and notice how many things are coming together for you. *Go to Section II to learn more (p 274).*

#99: This Too Will Pass (The Holographic Universe)

(5-6 minutes)

How to do SOS #99: This SOS method asks you to stop for a few minutes to gain a truly remarkable perspective. Whenever you feel yourself getting overwhelmed or stressed, just stop.

Use one of the Core breathing techniques to settle down. Then, when you feel centered, bring to mind the true nature of our holographic, constantly shifting Universe, i.e., *everything is always changing.* That makes it much easier whenever you're feeling bad to pause and remember: "This too shall pass."

The famous physicist David Bohm contended that whatever you're now experiencing is the *explicit* (visible) part of reality. This is what you can see, touch, feel, taste, smell, i.e., what *appears to be reality* at this moment. However, Bohm believed that there is infinitely more *implicit reality* (reality that is invisible, coming into or passing out of existence, and also reality that lies beyond the power of human perception). Truly, it is inevitable that your current problem will pass because that is the real nature of this dancing world in which you live.

So, for this SOS contemplation, simply pause to remember when this problem you're now having was *implicit* (did not yet exist or was not in your awareness)—and look beyond it now to the time when it too will pass. As Saint Teresa of Avila said less scientifically (but more poetically) than Bohm:

Let nothing trouble you. Let nothing bother you.

All things are passing, God never changes.

Patience obtains all things.

Whoever has God lacks nothing. God alone suffices.

Go to Section II to learn more (p 274).

#100: Get a Great Night's Sleep (Top 10 Tricks)

(6 seconds to 6 minutes)

How to do SOS #100: Choose one of the Top Ten Tricks below as a way to ensure a good night's sleep. Depending on which one you try, it will take 6 seconds to 6 minutes, so I've averaged these to be between 2-4 minutes.

The lack of sleep is a major health hazard of our stressful lifestyles. Twenty percent of Americans report getting less than 6 hours/night (significantly under the recommended 7-8 hours). And, we now know that sleep deprivation contributes to major health issues including heart problems, diabetes, obesity, depression, accidents, relationship difficulties, diminished learning and creative capacity, and lowered productivity. The hazards of sleep deprivation have become more widely recognized in recent years; for example, the Huffington Post has an entire section devoted to sleep issues—go to the Healthy Living tab or put "sleep" into the search box.

One of the big problems with stress is that it can launch a vicious cycle with your sleep: i.e., it can ruin one night's sleep, and then that lack of sleep causes more stress and dysfunction the next day, which in turn can ruin the next night's sleep. But here's SOS to the rescue with some tried-and-true tricks to help you get the solid night's sleep you desire.

Individually, any one of these SOS sleep-tricks can help you. Start by trying out one to replace a less functional habit that may be harming your sleep. Once that has become a new habit, experiment with others. By adopting a few of these easy techniques, you are guaranteed success. Below I have noted my Top Ten list; for rationale on how and why each of them works, go to Learn More. (BTW: Refer back to the 20-second rule to help you turn any one of these tricks into a new habit.)

1. Unplug! Turn off the TV or computer two hours (no less than one hour) before sleep time.

2. Do not watch the news within two hours of bedtime.

3. Have evening meal no closer than 3-4 hours before bedtime.

4. Spend quiet time with loved one(s) &/or call friends or family.

5. Prepare for the next day.

6. Parentheses (meditate or contemplate before & after sleep).

7. Eat a half-apple one to two hours before bedtime.

8. Soak, massage, or stretch out kinks in your body.

9. Design your own quiet time and place where you can relax.

10. Early to bed, early to rise (to be healthy, wealthy, and wise).

Go to Section II to learn more (p 276).

#101: Re-Balance with the Balance Beam

(Move from DisEase to Ease)

(4 minutes)

We conclude the Synergy section with the *Balance Beam*. You can use this tool to check your state of overall Ease, and then decide how to regain whatever ground you may have lost due to distress. *The Balancing Act assumes that your life is always in flux because you are always in the process of dealing with changing circumstances.* Balancing therefore is a *verb*, an on-going dynamic process of evolution and adaptation, stress and relaxation, balance and counterbalance, rather than a perfect (static) state to be achieved.

You can think of the *Balance Beam* as a gage that's designed to show why you're feeling in-balance or out-of-balance. It will also help you pinpoint whether this unease is because you are relying TOO MUCH on a particular element OR if you are paying TOO LITTLE attention to it. Both extremes can cause discomfort or dis-ease. The Balance Beam check-in will help you make course corrections so you do not derail completely.

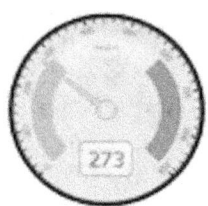

How to do SOS #101: Check all the descriptors that are true of you at this moment. With this feedback, you can decide how to bring yourself into better balance and greater ease. (For example, you can address that element directly, or you can look elsewhere for a root cause of this imbalance.)

Please Note: Do not be surprised if you have checks in opposite extremes of an element. This would indicate an element that is highly stressed and needs immediate attention. For example: in Mission, you could simultaneously feel apathetic and indecisive (in the first column) BUT you're in a workaholic state, running on fumes (in the third column). If so, it's no surprise that you're feeling so stressed.

COLUMN I (--) UNEASE to DISEASE Out of Balance: (Too little/underdeveloped)	COLUMN II (0) EASE – IN BALANCE	COLUMN III (+) UNEASE to DISEASE Out of Balance: (Overly reliant)
CORE (--)	CORE	CORE (+)
Take things too personally	Feel steady & calm	Detached; monkish
Weak self-esteem/confidence	Ethical, honest	Prefer to observe
Not aware of what feel/think	Strong self-esteem	Set self apart
Feel anxious much of time	Aware of thoughts	Passive; withdrawn

VISION (--)	VISION	VISION (+)
Afraid, fearful, anxious	Optimism, hope, positive	Cerebral/abstract
Pessimistic; negative	Inspired, creative	Thoughts loop
Hopeless, depressed	Good humor, fun	Jump from idea to next
Confused, unclear	Always learning	Hyper-critical

MISSION (--)	MISSION	MISSION (+)
Unclear goals, direction	Passionate, excited	Workaholic; push self
Low energy; burned-out	Disciplined, focused	Aggressive if pushed
Avoid conflict	Decisive; clear priorities	Win to prove worth
Slow to act or decide	Ambitious; proud	Burn candle-both ends

INTERACTIONS (--)	INTERACTIONS	INTERACTIONS (+)
Prefer to be alone	Welcoming, empathetic	Too emotional, moody
Detached, cool	Good listener, kind	Get involved in drama
Not demonstrative	Cooperate, build bridges	Defer to others
Do not suffer fools gladly	Healthy relationships	Manipulative

STRUCTURE (--)	STRUCTURE	STRUCTURE (+)
Impractical; unrealistic	Well-organized, reliable	Bureaucratic
Inefficient management	Effective; on time/task	Cautious, avoid errors
Dysfunctional habits	Responsible steward	Look to past for direction
Unrealistic goals	Good habits	Avoid change & risk

SYNERGY (--)	SYNERGY	SYNERGY (+)
Thrown off-balance	Holistic; see context	Miss details
Lack sense of whole	Feel luck, ease, gratitude	Magical thinking
Unlucky; blame others	Balanced, resilient, happy	Make tiny issues big
Lack resilience	Pragmatic; responsible	Inaction

Go to Section II to learn more (p 280).

SECTION II:

LEARN MORE ABOUT

THE 101 SOS TECHNIQUES

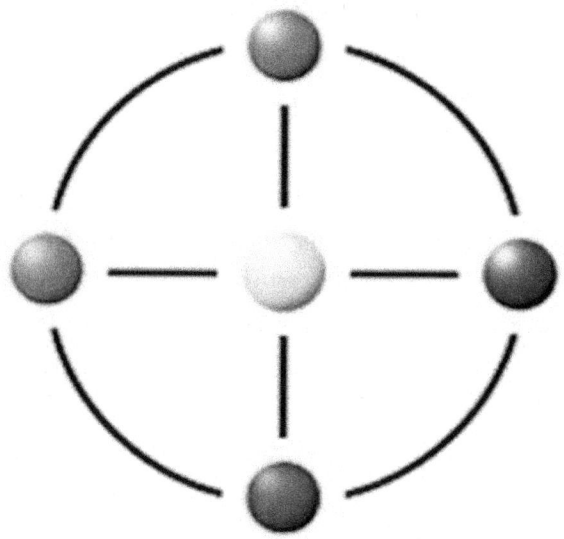

What the SOS techniques can do for you.

Why they work.

Where you can discover more.

This Section of SOS is a rich resource center for learning more about any SOS technique you particularly like.

Learn More about SOS CORE Techniques

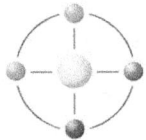

To discover how the Core element can move you from stress to success, please read the Core description that begins SOS Chapter One, Section I. You can also read the Core chapter in *The Balancing Act* (pages 35-48) to see how this element affects your life, relationships and work. (To read more about TBA go to http://balance.thecoreporation.com.)

#1: Experience the Calming Core Element

Learn more about SOS #1: The Core audio is an abbreviated version of a "progressive relaxation". This is a powerful process in which you consciously release, from head to toe, all the tension you may be holding in your body that prevents you from being relaxed and in touch with your Core. For a longer version of a good progressive relaxation, go to "feature=player_detailpage&v=2ZKNr-W9A1U".

#2: Stealth Breath

Learn more about SOS #2: Most of us breathe shallowly most of the time. This is actually very bad for our health. And this tendency only increases when we perceive an active threat and move into a knee-jerk stress reaction of fight or flight. I use all the Core breathing techniques as conscious *neuro-interruptors*—i.e., they keep the normal neurological stress reflex patterns from continuing unabated by providing a priceless instant during which you can stop excessive stress signals. In effect, all these deep breathing Core techniques countermand your stress response by saying: "All's well…it's a false alarm…you can bring the troops back home now".

Here's why Core breathing is important. When you inhale, your lungs expand as the air passes through them, to your alveoli (air sacs), and from there to your blood cells. Your heart then pumps oxygen-rich blood throughout your body. At the same time as your heart is pumping oxygen to all the places your body needs it, it is also moving carbon dioxide from the blood vessels to the alveoli through your lungs—and finally out of your body through your nose or mouth.

By exhaling carbon dioxide, you release impurities, toxins and stress from your body. With each breath, you have a healthier ration of oxygen to carbon dioxide; this is why breathing deeply makes you feel calmer, healthier and rejuvenated.

Research indicates that deep breathing has myriad positive impacts on your health. These include strengthening the following internal systems: respiratory, digestive, lymph, circulatory, immune, nervous, and cleansing. It also helps heal muscles and joints, reduces mental and physical pain, improves mental clarity, decision-making, physical appearance, and strengthens spirituality, intuition, creativity, and relationships. (And if that wasn't enough, deep breathing even acts as a natural aphrodisiac—now do I have your attention?)

So with this information in mind, every time you notice that you're breathing shallowly, reset by taking a deep breath and become a "stealth breather" instead. Once you've mastered this basic technique, you may want to expand your practice. If so, read this excellent article: yogajournal.com/practice/1523.

#3: Walking Breath

Learn more about SOS #3: Because so many of my clients find it difficult at first to just-sit-still-and-breathe, I have them start their centering practices while in motion. (True confessions: this is how I began managing my own stress when I was the CEO of Central Minnesota Group Health Plan. I thought it was a great *two-for-the price-of-one* activity because while I walked to work, I could simultaneously exercise AND meditate.)

Almost invariably, clients who are most resistant to taking any quiet time-out (but who agree to do the walking breath), wind up reporting how much this technique helps them improve their athleticism. They're soon able to do more laps in the pool, run longer distances, have more endurance during tennis games, etc. After these unanticipated happy outcomes, conscious Core breathing becomes a new, valued part of the fabric of their lives. It's usually not long before they notice other, more subtle benefits—and are finally willing and able to just-sit-still-and-breathe for a few moments.

By adding the breath count to your steps, you will likely enjoy the walk more because you're paying attention to your body and your surroundings. Rather than worrying about what's next, you'll be able to stay in the here-and-now, and you'll walk more gracefully while also avoiding those real bumps in the road.

Just try it. At first the walking breath count is a bit like trying to rub your stomach while patting your head at the same time. But soon it becomes a relief—and finally a pleasure—to glide along to your destination rather than push yourself forward. Go to Learn More SOS #2 to see research about breathing benefits.

#4: Emergency Breath

Learn more about SOS #4: This technique instantly interrupts the stress cycle. Much like using dynamite to blast a boulder out of the way for a new railroad track, this activity removes mental boulders, thereby allowing you to lay new neurological tracks that will get you quickly to your new habits.

After doing the Emergency Breath, you will likely feel incredibly invigorated. I encourage you to do it several times a day (in private, because it's noisy and I don't want you to become the subject of ridicule). This is a phenomenal stress-buster—fast and easy to do many times a day no matter how busy you are.

The mental and physical benefits of repeating this technique regularly are numerous. They include: increased pulmonary capacity (directly tied to longevity), cardiovascular system improvement, detoxification (full release of carbon dioxide), plus improved lymphatic and immune system functioning.

#5: Soothing Sounds

Learn more about SOS #5: Of the 5 senses, *sound* is the one associated with your Essence or Core. Numerous studies have shown the healing effects of certain kinds of music for the human heart, immune system, mental health, speed of healing recovery, and general well being.

Unfortunately, many of us are bombarded almost constantly with *noise*—unhealthy sounds that permeate modern life (background traffic, sirens, the persistent hum of home and work machinery, video games, TV ads or programs, people speaking loudly on their cell phones, etc.). Noise pollution is now widely recognized as a health hazard. Not only does it adversely affect our hearing, but it is also a major contributor to sleep disorders, problems with concentration, fatigue, feelings of irritation, decreased work productivity, disturbed interpersonal relationships, and other stress reactions.

When you choose silence or these soothing sounds for just a few minutes, you will feel more at ease. I experience an almost-instant relief, like a temporary cease-fire of the ongoing assault on my mind and body: my muscles relax, I can breathe more easily and deeply, and my mind stays quiet long enough so I can actually produce an original thought!

Interestingly, soothing sounds are life-giving not just for human beings, but also for all living organisms. There is a famous experiment that demonstrates how plants grow TOWARD speakers broadcasting classical music and AWAY from speakers playing hard rock music. This experiment showed that plants prefer instrumental classical Western music of 60 beats per second (the resting human heart rate) and classical music from India, where the musical scale is tuned to a slower vibration. The implications are significant for your health if you, like most of us, are inundated with constant-noise-and-stimuli. Please give yourself a break by substituting SOS (and other) Soothing Sounds for ongoing noise bombardment.

#6: Small Universe

Learn more about SOS #6: This is a variation of a Qigong sitting meditation that is taught by Dr. Chunyi Lin of Spring Forest Qigong. Dr. Lin is a world-renown healer with his own school of Tai Chi. I love to do this exercise first thing in the morning. I also have found that it is wonderful to do when I am walking out doors, or when I need an energy boost or to quiet my anxiety, rebalance and center myself.

To find out more about Dr. Lin's excellent stress reducing techniques, visit Learningstrategies.com. I have taken Dr. Lin's

Level 1 and 2 training, and recommend anything he teaches if you wish to take further steps to Switch Off Stress.

#7: Countdown

Learn more about SOS #7: These countdown techniques are so pervasive that I cannot remember where I first experienced them. Although countdowns like this one have been used in hypnotic processes for as long as these have existed, in more recent decades they've also been used to support a myriad of self-help relaxation techniques.

One famous version of the 3-2-1 count down is the Silva Centering Technique. In the Silva system the "3" level is for deep physical relaxation, the "2" level is for deep mental relaxation, and the "1" level is for powerful whole-brain actualization. After you program yourself with this centering technique, whenever you repeat the 3-2-1 command, your system will respond with deepened relaxation.

Go to silvamethod.com to learn about Jose Silva and the organization he founded. You can get a free "starter kit" course there if you would like to explore this groundbreaking work and/or have Laura Silva (daughter of Jose) guide you through a 30 minute "3-2-1" Silva Centering Meditation. You can also watch "feature=player_detailpage& v=05TwQ6OYXW0". (Note: you can skip the 4½-minute introduction if you choose.)

#8: Access Your GPS

Learn more about SOS #8: Here's why you should you use your internal GPS…. Much as a car's GPS can access a worldwide internet with its extraordinary wealth of expertise and intelligence (thousands of map makers and satellite engineers, etc.), your intuition benefits from millions of information signals that bombard your senses every second of your life.

Although your Mind's pre-programed perceptual filters are able to process 16 bits of (what the Mind considers to be) relevant information every second, your intuition processes an extraordinary wash of <u>11 million bits of information per second</u>! See landmark research detailed in *The User Illusion: Cutting Consciousness Down to Size* by Danish science writer Tor Norretranders, where he argues that our hunches are much closer to "reality" than what our minds tell us. It is this wealth of GPS-like accessible data that makes intuitive intelligence a preferred avenue for complex decision-making. (That's true for all of us, but even more so for our often-beleaguered leaders who are wrestling daily with high-impact, mind-boggling problems.) Intuition also helps us access "flashes" of memory from our personal data banks that we've stored but forgotten.

We often refer to our hunches as *gut instincts*. (Interestingly, in some Chinese healing systems, the nerve-rich gut is referred to as our *second brain*.) Many philosophers and most indigenous cultures argue that much of the knowledge of human history and wisdom is available through our instincts. They say that, as animals, we have an extraordinary bank of information encoded in our DNA—and that, much as geese know how to fly south for winter, we too have a *collective unconscious* (a term coined by Carl Jung's) at our beck and call to guide us safely…if only we stop, tune in, and listen.

#9: Sing those Blues Away

Learn more about SOS #9: Since ancient times, across all cultures, singing and chanting have been considered healing tools. Singing influences brain wave frequencies and promotes wellbeing. It can reduce stress and improve mood; lower blood pressure; boost the immune system; improve breathing; reduce perceived pain; promote learning and increase memory.

Singing necessitates deep breathing, an anxiety reducer. It produces effects similar to exercise, including the release of endorphins, the body's feel-good hormones. This gives the singer an overall "lifted" feeling. (Now karaoke makes a lot more sense, doesn't it?) Singing is actually an aerobic activity, getting more oxygen into the blood for better circulation—which in turn contributes to a better mood. Singing also vibrates your body from the inside out, "tuning" it to increased happiness.

If you have children, encourage them to sing just for the fun of it and/or to help them deal with the blues. In older cultures, EVERYONE sang as a natural part of daily life, and there were songs for all occasions. Reclaim this wonderful part of your human heritage both for yourself and for those you love. Lift your voice and recapture that sheer joy.

And lastly, if you're stressed by political or social injustices, singing is a time-tested way to create solidarity and confront external obstacles without violence. As the New Song movement (*Canto Nuevo*) in South America and the Civil Rights movement in America emphasized: "you can't have a revolution without songs".

And here, as promised, are the lyrics to "*Don't Worry, Be Happy*" and "Happy" (see also 24hoursofhappy.com):

*Here's a little song I wrote, you might want to sing it note for note –
Don't worry, be happy*

*In every life we have some trouble, But when you worry you make it
double -- Don't worry, be happy. (Repeat)*

*Ain't got no place to lay your head, Somebody came and took your bed --
Don't worry, be happy.*

*The landlord say your rent is late, He may have to litigate --
Don't worry, be happy. (Repeat)*

It might seem crazy what I'm about to say,
Sunshine she's here, you can take a break.
I'm a hot air balloon that could go to space
With the air, like I don't care baby, by the way...because I'm happy.

(Chorus): Clap along if you feel like a room without a roof.
Clap along if you feel like happiness is the truth.
Clap along if you know what happiness is to you.
Clap along if you feel like that's what you wanna do.

Here come bad news talking this and that, yeah,
Well, give me all you got, and don't hold it back.
Well, I should probably warn you, I'll be just fine.
No offense to you, don't waste your time. (Chorus)

188

#10: Beam Me Up

Learn more about SOS #10: This exercise has been used in various forms ever since humanity first looked up, noticed the sun in the sky, and felt its rays seeping in to warm and relax the whole body. I have seen variations of this activity done in many cultures and healing traditions.

Christie Marie Sheldon does a great version of this exercise in her "Love or Above" course (see christiesheldon.com).

#11: Lightning Strikes

Learn more about SOS #11: The Magician archetype is said to gain healing energy by drawing down the powers of heaven and drawing up the powers of earth, so they meet halfway in the healer's heart. (Which is why Magicians are often shown as having one arm pointed up and the other pointed down.)

Interestingly, the Magician image mimics the phenomenon of cloud-to-ground lightning; the lighting explosions we see are the manifestation of the attraction of electrical potential between positive and negative charges. These charges eventually grow strong enough to overcome the air's resistance to electrical flow. Racing toward each other, the charges connect, completing an electrical circuit, and discharging the accumulated electricity as lightning. Although you likely won't experience this SOS exercise as a bolt of lightning, you should feel much stronger and powerful as a result.

If you wish to learn more about the Magician archetype, go to thecoreporation.com to read summaries of the Magician and other Core Types or take a free quiz on this website to learn about your preferences among the ten heroic Core Types.

You can also read *Working from Your Core* to learn how to access the advice of these 10 different kinds of heroes.

#12: Breathe a Smile In – Breathe Toxins Out

Learn more about SOS #12: See commentary on the health benefits of breathing by reviewing the notes in Learn More about SOS #2. Then you can review the extensive research on the health benefits of smiling in Learn More about SOS #58.

#13: Call a Time Out

Learn more about SOS #13: Whenever you take a break, you're hitting the refresh button on yourself. You're stepping back and starting over with a clear mind and better attitude. You're getting ready to make the winning goal. Also, you're redoing the concept of time-out by switching these breaks into fun—and making them a normal, welcome part of your day.

Recent research indicates that businesses would be well advised to encourage employees to take breaks during working hours. Successful companies such as Google, Facebook and LinkedIn have instituted as much as 20% "time-out" to increase innovation. (These policies have led to huge wildly profitable inventions such as Gmail and AdSense; see more at: "cnn.com/2014/05/16/opinion/schulte-daydreaming-productivity/".

Prior research suggests that taking a short break every 60-90 minutes is necessary to maintain focus (other researchers argue for a break every 45 minutes). What we know for certain is that the longer people are on duty, the less accurate reporting becomes. People need to regularly reset their ability to focus. The most effective time-out is to shift attention by doing something completely different from your work. For most white-collar workers, this would be some activity that does not engage the brain. For blue-collar workers, a refreshing break may mean picking up a good book. The advantage of taking intermittent short breaks is that it's a way of respecting our natural body rhythms. When we take short times-out, we can reduce stress that's silently building up, then return to our tasks feeling refreshed, relaxed and re-inspired.

Often work breaks mean snacking down on sugary food to get a quick pick-me-up. In SOS you'll find other suggestions. For example, eat food that will give your brain and energy a strong boost (see SOS #84) or have a cup of tea (see SOS #78). Doing some exercises or stretching can be a good idea too (See SOS #42 and SOS #44.) Get some fresh air. Take a moment to chat with a friend or colleague. Time-outs like these improve our quality of life and help us regain perspective.

As Tony Schwartz, CEO of The Energy Project, states in the Harvard Business Review Blog Network: (http://blogs.hbr.org/2011/12/how-to-accomplish-more-by-doin/) "Human beings are designed to pulse rhythmically between spending and renewing energy. That's how we operate at our best. Maintaining a steady reservoir of energy — physically, mentally, emotionally and even spiritually—requires refueling it intermittently." So…do it! Take a time out.

#14: No More Waiting to Exhale

Learn more about SOS #14: The health benefits of exhalation are vastly underrated. Most of us know that we release impurities by exhaling carbon dioxide. However, did you know that *we expel about 75 percent of our body's natural toxins during exhalation?* (WOW! What are you waiting for?)

Exhalation is not only great for your body; it's also an effective way to quickly grab hold of your emotions before they hijack you. Deep exhalation immediately improves your mood while simultaneously calming, reenergizing and balancing your mind. Don't wait to exhale! By doing so you eliminate toxins, increase feelings of relaxation, relieve stress, free your respiratory system so it can inhale more fresh air, and move fresh oxygen throughout your whole body.

I now prefer the "3/5" shorter inhale/longer exhale breath count vs. the evenly balanced 4/4 count. According to proponents, the 3/5 breath mimics our deep relaxation and natural sleeping

breath. To learn more, read: myyogaonline.com/about-yoga/
pranayama/yoga-breathing-for-health.

#15: Talk to Your Smartest Self

Learn more about SOS #15: These instructions are based on a powerful contemplative technique I learned many years ago from a Siddha Yoga monk, Swami Umeshananda. I had a breakthrough understanding the very first time I tried it, and have continued to use this self-dialogue process throughout the years. I have passed on this technique to my clients, many of whom have benefited from it mightily over the years.

To learn more about why your "in-tuition" can offer you such remarkably smart, unexpected, breakthrough answers to your most puzzling problems, go to Learn More about SOS #8.

#16: Make a Space around the Pain

Learn more about SOS #16: If you'd like to learn more and expand your practice of either of these techniques, please go to the following resources. The Option One technique is a simplified version of the Sedona Method. (Go to sedona.com to learn more about this excellent work.) You can test drive this powerful method for releasing anxiety by watching a 2-minute demonstration of one very easy Sedona technique (feature=player_detailpage&v=2jEtTublJYM).

The Option Two technique is derived from stories in Eckhart Tolle's *A New Earth* (from *Chapter Six: Breaking Free*). Go to eckharttolle.com to find many helpful videos, books and courses that will further your stress relief practices.

#17: Sounds and Silence

Learn more about SOS #17: Deliberately putting yourself in an Observer role is an excellent way to set yourself apart from whatever is causing you anxiety so you can relax and regain your internal balance.

In this SOS technique we have focused on the sense of hearing, because sound is the sense associated with the Core element. However, you can modify this activity by focusing on the other senses in a similar fashion. For example, you can gaze at a beautiful scene, focusing your eyes on just one tree in a stand. Notice all the details about it. Make it the foreground, as if you were an artist deciding your perspective for a painting. Then shift your visual focus to something else, perhaps a leaf that's fallen on the ground, or a wild flower. Similarly you can focus on different tastes while you are eating, different textures you are touching, etc.

Learn More about SOS VISION Techniques

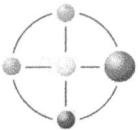

To discover how Vision can move you from stress to success, please read the Vision element description that begins SOS Chapter Two, Section I. You can also read the Vision chapter in *The Balancing Act* (pages 68-84) to see how this element affects your life, relationships and work. (To read more about TBA go to http://balance.thecoreporation.com.)

#18: Experience the Inspiring Element of Vision

Learn more about SOS #18: Another simple, but powerful visioning activity is this two-part exercise. Take four minutes in the morning: a) two minutes to envision your ideal life 3-5 years in the future, and then b) two minutes to imagine what you would like to do today to bring this ideal dream closer to reality.

When visioning try to use all 5 senses to make this experience as "real" as possible: see colors, touch objects you imagine in your mind's eye, notice sounds and smells if at all possible. I find that using soothing sounds (SOS#5) or meditation music in the background keeps me focused while I'm visioning.

Other excellent visioning activities include creating a Vision Board or a personal PowerPoint presentation with images of the life you want. You could also watch or create short Mind

Movies. (You can get several free Mind Movies and discover how to make your own by visiting mindmovies.com.)

Keep in mind that visioning can take the short range, detailed, granular perspective of a mouse, or the long range soaring sky-wide vision of an eagle. (People who are Myers Briggs Type "Sensors" tend to prefer the former, while MBTI "Intuitives" may prefer the latter). Start with whichever kind of visioning makes the most sense to you and then try the other perspective as well, because each visioning approach has different benefits.

#19: STOP IT!

Learn more about SOS #19: Don't allow your mind to run (or ruin) your life. Unfortunately, left to its own devises your Mind is likely to be critical—particularly of you. Repetitive thoughts are very rarely in the "you're the tops" category; they're much more likely to be some variation of "You screwed up again, you idiot".

Many meditation traditions refer to our lack of mental control as _monkey mind_—relentless noisy chattering as the mind swings like an agitated monkey from tree limb to tree limb. The happy alternative to this exhausting and debilitating mental state comes from mental control and discipline. _The Balancing Act_ process ensures that your Mind is directed by your Core (values, identity, gifts)—for your sake and everyone else's.

"Stopping it" helps you align your Mind with your Core. This simple step is akin to stopping so you can put a skilled driver behind the steering wheel of a powerful car. Not only is it safer for everyone in the car and on the road, it also makes it more likely you will arrive safely at the destination you've envisioned.

#20: Take a Laughter Break

Learn more about SOS #20: Laughter is truly the best medicine; it has been healing humanity for millennia and can pop a stress-bubble faster than anything. And it has many of the same health benefits as a good workout: increased blood flow, strengthened immune system, improved mood, lowered blood sugar, and pain relief—to name just a few. (Read these articles: webmd.com/balance/features/give-your-body-boost-with-laughter; mayoclinic.org/healthy-living/stress-management/in-depth/stress-relief/art-20044456 and http://stress.about.com/od/stresshealth/a/laughter.htm. You can also go to SOS #60 to learn about Laughter Yoga.)

There is even an archetype whose special cure for distress is laughter: the Jester. (An archetype is a natural human instinct, which means that you have a Jester part of yourself just waiting to get out.) The really smart Rulers of yore had Jesters in their courts to tell them any truth the yes-men wouldn't dare to voice. Jesters also consider it their duty to pop the bubble of over-seriousness and pomposity that can blind Rules from seeing the best solutions.

Today we find remarkable Jesters in some of the world's hot spots: just look to the political comic movement sweeping the

Middle East, including Bassem Youssef, the "Jon Stewart of Egypt", and Saudi comics Hisham Fageeh and Fahad al-Butairi whose "No Woman, No Drive" became a viral sensation: feature=player_detailpage&v=aZMbTFNp4wI. These are just a few examples of the many other careful-but-courageous comics throughout the world. God bless you, one and all—you are the heroic Jesters of our time! (You can read more about the Jester Core Type at thecoreporation.com or get *Working from Your Core*, in which a whole chapter is devoted to the Jester.)

One of the great things about funny videos is that it's so easy to share a laugh in an instant. Here are some videos that made me laugh out loud: Baby & Beyonce (v=9yEtf-r08uM); Twins & Daddy's Guitar (v=to7uIG8KYhg); Funny Cats (v=nTasT5h0Leg); Dog & Baby (v=Q5QvylbPyvc). Enjoy!

Happily for all of us, there are entertaining videos, movies and programs being created every day, so rest assured that you and your internal Jester will never run out of material to enjoy on your laughter breaks.

#21: Slow Down Your Brain Waves

Learn more about SOS #21: Human beings have a wide range of brain wave states. If you want to become the smartest and most effective person you can possibly be, here is a rough approximation of major brain wave ranges: *Delta* (0.5-4 HZ, deep sleep); *Theta* (4-8 HZ, deep meditation and relaxation); *Alpha* (relaxed awake state, 8-13 HZ); and *Beta* (13-30, awake

198

and active). Experience examples of all these wave states by inputting key words in YouTube or by going to SOS #21 at thecoreporation.com/sos_links.

Most relaxation and meditation exercises focus on getting you to the alpha state; this is about **10** brain cycles per second. Alpha is a relatively emotion-and-stress-free state where you do your best thinking, make optimal decisions, and learn.

When you're awake (beta) the ideal brainwave frequency would be approximately **20** cycles per second. Beta is where we live, work and play most of the time; it is also the world of emotions.

Unfortunately, the more you like or dislike something, the more emotional you become. This raises your brain wave frequency to above 30. When you are in the grip of elevated brain-wave states, you feel overwhelmed. What's worse, you become less capable of thinking clearly. When anger turns into rage, or fear into panic, brain waves can rise above 30. Here you use very little of your mind. You no longer consider consequences, and this is when stress can cause real trouble. People who are enraged can strike out violently; panicked people can drown because they don't swim toward a life raft.

All this suffering happens when brain waves rise so steeply that people's minds shut down. So next time you notice that your thinking is getting out of control, use SOS activities to slow down your brain waves so you don't become a statistic.

#22: The Tetris Effect

Learn more about SOS #22: I recommended that you read *The Happiness Advantage,* where author Shawn Anchor dedicates a whole chapter to using the Tetris Effect so it increases your happiness. Check it out—you'll love the book.

The Tetris Effect is a common human phenomenon where you scan for patterns—these can be positive, negative or neutral. For example, a neutral effect is when you see white cars everywhere after you've decided to buy one. In truth, we have thousands of perceptual filters that probably operate us more than we operate them. It is worth stepping back and observing if you might be using perceptual filters that hamper you in any way. This takes vigilance, curiosity and the courage first, to tell yourself the truth—and second, to make changes if required. A block for most of us is that we think our worldview is right, and our filters constantly "prove" and reinforce our perspectives, whether we start out as Scrooge or Pollyanna.

It's up to you to observe, then decide upon the balance and clarity you'd like to have as your daily operating perceptual system—and then counterbalance the power of any dysfunctional Tetris Effect by deliberately putting a more functional lens into action. (See Shawn Anchor's lively video lecture: feature=player_detailpage&v=ae-ypgdd5-8.)

To adjust your Tetris Effect and reframe your daily dose of news, check out alternate "good news" sites: dailygood.org; goodnewsnetwork.org; huffingtonpost.com/goodnews.

#23: Get Inspired

Learn more about SOS #23: This is another way to reframe the Tetris Effect, i.e., you deliberately focus your mind on the positive (almost like tuning an instrument to a higher vibration, or finding the right radio station on the dial.)

Here's a great web site to launch you in the practice of regularly reading inspirational quotes: quotery.com/top-100-inspirational-quotes-of-all-time. Just pick a quote to start your day, savor it in the moment—and then save it for easy reference. Here's one that suits the Vision element well: *The best way to predict the future is to invent it* (Alan Kay). You could start your own "favorite quotes" personal file, or program a quote-of-the-day to be your computer's screen saver.

You can do a similar "get-inspired" process with beautiful images. Find a photo book (for example of a travel destination) and pick a stunning image. If you want to use the computer to do the same thing, you can put your keyword into a search engine and see what visuals pop up. And if you want to store your inspiring images, you can create a Vision board or use Pinterest, WeHeartIt, or similar visual sites.

You can also build a library of inspiring books that you keep close at hand in your office or home for the moment you need inspiration. Or, you could put eBooks you like on your eReader, notepad, or computer so you can have them immediately at hand. (I hope SOS becomes one of them!) And of course, I encourage you to fill your music systems with uplifting songs that are ready for you whenever you need them.

This SOS technique is a counterbalancing force that lifts us up so we can see, reach, hear, and touch the stars, including meeting the minds of luminaries who have walked—and still walk—among us. I hope you embrace the inspiration you find and pass it on to others who would appreciate that support.

#24: Time Travel (Anticipation & Memories)

Learn more about SOS #24: Many physicists and mathematicians in the past decades have echoed the long-time assertion of meditators and old religions/philosophies that modern Western civilization's concepts of time and space are largely illusions. Although it's a bit mind-bending to even contemplate, some of these cutting-edge thinkers and researchers argue that all time is "now", and that the past and the future actually exist in the present. Although this debate about the reality of time and space is unlikely to be resolved anytime soon, we can use this challenge to the static definition of reality to help us reduce our stress in the here-and-now.

A great example of positive and negative anticipation is going on vacation. People typically experience excitement as they think about their coming weeks off. It's almost as good as already being there. But then, a few days before traveling home people start anticipating all the work they have to do when they return—and *even though they're still on vacation*, their minds are back in the office, dealing with problems that await them.

Knowing how the Mind perceives time gives you an edge—you can catch yourself as you're slipping into worry about something that has NOT yet occurred and also prevent yourself from getting lost in regrets about the past. Instead, you can transform remembering into a gratitude exercise and anticipation into a stress-reducing problem-solving tool. That is, by anticipating what the situation might be like and preparing for best ways to handle it, you'll do a mental dress rehearsal that helps you manage the situation well when the time arrives. (As long as you don't repeatedly loop this mental rehearsal.)

Numerous studies over the last 30 years have shown how our treatment of memories affects our life satisfaction. One study found that people's views about the past, present and future (i.e., their take on "What really happened…") determines their happiness. Another study showed that savoring happy memories and reframing painful past experiences in a positive light were particularly effective ways for individuals to increase their life satisfaction.

#25: Mirror of the Mind

Learn more about SOS #25: The Mirror of the Mind exercise is a great activity, used for the past decades by untold numbers of individuals to improve their lives. I hope you enjoy the below-listed audio by Laura Silva (head of the Silva organization and daughter of founder, Jose Silva). The Silva organization generously allows people to download this audio to use again and again. Go here for link to "Mirror of the Mind": silvalifesystem.com/exclusive/exercises/mirror-of-the-mind#sthash.37ql2OAH.dpbs.

#26: C'mon, Get Happy!

Learn more about SOS #26: Tom Robbins in *Still Life with Woodpecker* famously stated that: "It's never too late to have a happy childhood". As it turns out, rose-tinted glasses and a glass-half-full philosophy of life are actually healthy perspectives (as long as you avoid denial or lying to yourself).

We now know that it is WAY healthier to be happy than to be sad. Martin Seligman, who is credited with founding the field of Positive Psychology (Thank you, good sir!), says there are seven key factors for happiness. These are: your relationships, caring for others, exercise, flow (working toward a meaningful goal), spiritual engagement and meaning, using your strengths in your life, and having a positive mindset. (In this list there's no mention of "I won the lottery" or "I'm SO famous" or "I get paid more than you do". Surprised?)

I recommend that you visit Martin Seligman's website: pursuit-of-happiness.org to check out the Happiness Project. You can also visit www.Happier.com to get yourself a smart phone app so you can easily track the three happy things that happen to you every day. With this Happiness app, you can also share (and multiply) your happiness with others. This is truly a great way to spread sunshine all over the place.

And for extra fun, you can blast out your stress with these videos and the below sing-along lyrics (by Harold Arlen & Ted Koehler) to the classic song *C'mon, Get Happy!* Choose your artist and enjoy:

- Ella Fitzgerald (v=mwoPIRR9J_k)

- Judy Garland (v=2U-rBZREQMw)

- Katie Holmes (v=SdW4xVhsnhY)

Forget your troubles, Come on get happy,

You better chase all your cares away.

Shout hallelujah, Come on get happy!

Get ready for the judgment day.

The sun is shining, Come on get happy.

The lord is waiting to take your hand.

Shout hallelujah, Come on get happy.

We're going to the Promised Land.

We're heading cross the river.

Wash your sins away in the tide.

It's all so peaceful on the other side…. (Repeat.)

#27: How Much Will this Matter in...?

Learn more about SOS #27: When we're wrapped up in our problems, they can carry us away to utter exhaustion and feeling overwhelmed. However, if you stop to *reframe* any stressful situation with this no-nonsense question, you'll make better choices because you'll have a more objective perspective with which to reconsider your current problem.

When I was struggling to launch Central Minnesota Group Health Plan (and in a hurry pretty much all of the time), I had an easy-going friend, Joe Felix, who went even further than these questions. He would suggest the "Ice Age" test, i.e., "Will what you're doing matter in the next Ice Age?" Although this challenge was stated humorously, it always forced me to admit that all this drama was unimportant in the long run—and even less important when viewed from the Ice Age perspective!

#28: How Did You Contribute to This?

Learn more about SOS #28: The philosophy of Pragmatism urges constant experimentation in the laboratory of our daily lives so we can learn what does and does not work well—and why. Pragmatism assumes that mistakes are a natural part of our learning process. Stopping to complain and blame only slows the process of intelligent course correction. Charles Sanders Pierce (the "father" of Pragmatism) believed that real-life learning and experimentation was the ONLY way we could discover how we needed to adapt and evolve.

Pragmatism bases the meaning of things on their practical impact in action. Both *The Balancing Act* and *SOS: Switch Off Stress* are deeply rooted in pragmatism—which has helped our clients increase their resilience, meet and overcome major challenges, and manage change in shifting environments.

Pragmatism holds that "to believe something is to be willing to act on it". The basic components of pragmatic logic include a) preparing for successful action based on current beliefs, and b) *improving beliefs* based on the results of past actions. Intelligence, according to pragmatism, aims for sustainable successful results, plus ongoing learning and adaptation. (Here adaptation is defined as "having a capacity to make fit for new or special situations; flexible; a successful adjustment".)

The development of philosophical Pragmatism contributed directly to the business practices of quality improvement. The PDCA Cycle (Plan, Do, Check, Act) was designed by Walter Shewhart and popularized by his most famous student, W. Edwards Deming. Their work comes directly from the intellectual lineage of the American pragmatists, which include John Dewey, William James, C. I. Lewis, E. A. Singer, and C. S. Peirce. Furthermore, many of the most critical business management philosophies of the late 20th century (TQM, knowledge management, action learning, organization learning) are rooted in the work of these early American pragmatists.

#29: Mental Shielding

Learn more about SOS #29: Here are some real-life examples of successes I've seen with this unusual technique. One of my clients who had a hypercritical, humiliating boss chose to imagine Power Rangers beside her during their discussions; she even put several of these toys on her office desk to remind her of her Power Ranger alter ego! It was all she could do to not laugh out loud whenever she saw her secret back-up team. Interestingly, the boss lightened up soon thereafter, for no apparent reason. (I'm guessing it was a positive response to my client's lighter interactions.)

Another client, a physician, selected as her shield a magical membrane much like the Native American dream web (which supposedly allows in good dreams and keeps out nightmares). This mental picture helped her keep the nastiness of her misogynist boss outside this imaginary membrane while allowing in the support of her political allies. She also had the smarts to take a further step: she allowed only her own positive thoughts/feelings out of her membrane so that she would not adversely affect others when she was feeling stressed. I was quite impressed. She not only transformed her own attitude, but she also managed to survive the tenure of that manager and got a much better new boss instead.

I've had one client use an "invisibility cloak" to stay out of the way of a difficult co-worker. Another chose the mental picture of a Chernobyl-like nuclear protection suit for her incredibly hostile workplace. She'd take a few moments to "suit-up" completely in her mind before she set foot in the lobby. These imaging exercises made these two feel safer and be productive while gaining confidence to make fast tracks for departure.

The Mind is so powerful that you can use this exercise as a way to deliberately trick yourself into feeling more safe and stable. Of course, this tool is not to be used to deny real danger, but rather to control environments where your mind is perhaps imagining more danger than is true—and also to control and calm your subtle contributions to these difficulties. For example, you may decide to use this technique to reduce the potential damage in a situation: yes, that person may dislike you, but you've taken action to shield yourself from his bad thoughts or comments. That way, you'll experience less of his negativity "getting through" your shielding. This, after all, is what shields are designed to do—i.e., to protect you from harm.

There are many traditions throughout the world that have called upon the power of the mind for protection. Even today, many sci-fi traditions (novels, movies, video games) use mental shielding for their super-powered heroes. What we're proposing in this SOS technique is something much more simple, light-hearted and good-natured for daily use so can do your part to transform negative situations into more positive ones.

#30: Subliminal Stress Relief

Learn more about SOS #30: Go to richarluck.com for details of how this innovative system was developed. You may also want to check out the below video, which explains Luck's technology and products, while also providing a free demo to improve your self-confidence (subliminal-videos.com/ty21/thankyou.php? track =newblogbanner).

#31: Reframe Stress as a Friend and Teacher

Learn more about SOS #31: To quote William Shakespeare: "Thinking makes it so." It is a major premise of _SOS: Switch Off Stress_ that thinking of stress as an ally can transform into a friend or pragmatic teacher—so I won't belabor the point here. The questions noted in this exercise are the kinds that will allow you to follow the symptoms of stress to their root causes. And, in turn, that will allow you to do something about the originating problems so they are less likely to recur.

#32: Give Your Eyes a Break

Learn more about SOS #32: Concentrated use of the eyes is stressful. And eyestrain, in turn, causes more stress on the rest of your body. Without breaks like the ones suggested in this SOS technique, you could experience symptoms such as ocular fatigue, blurring, headaches, dry eyes, and double vision. Concentrating on reading fine print or using the computer for hours at a time can make you unconsciously clench the muscles of your eyelids, face, temples, and jaws, then cause discomfort or pain from overusing those muscles. This may lead to a vicious cycle of tensing those muscles further and causing even more toxic stress and tiredness.

Common precipitating factors for eyestrain include extended use of a computer or video monitor, straining to see in very dim light, and exposure to extreme brightness or glare. Many people will blink less than normal when performing extended visual tasks. This decreased blinking may lead to dryness of the ocular surface (dry eyes). Happily, many of these problems can be prevented easily by taking regular visual breaks.

#33: Participant/Observer Dual Lens

Learn more about SOS #33: I've seen variations of this SOS technique taught in numerous traditions, but I began to practice it after I took the *Crack your Egg* course designed by Henk Schram. For more information about Schram's excellent work, go to http://crackyoureggprogram.com/ where you will find free videos and PDF instructions so you can sample this terrific program.

#34: Observe, Ask, Learn, Adapt

Learn more about SOS #34: This technique is another approach to treating distress with a logical, pragmatic, action-learning approach.

Go to Learn More about SOS #28 to read about pragmatism and action learning. There you will also see how pragmatism relates to *The Balancing Act, SOS: Switch Off Stress*, and why a pragmatic approach improves the odds of your making lasting improvements in your life, relationships and work.

———————————————

Learn More about SOS MISSION Techniques

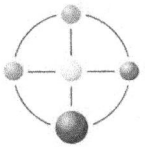

To discover how Mission can move you from stress to success, please read the Mission element description that begins SOS Chapter Three, Section I. You can also read the Mission chapter in *The Balancing Act* (pages 100-111) to see how this element affects your life, relationships and work. (Go to http://balance.thecoreporation.com to read more about TBA.)

#35: Experience the Motivating Element of Mission

Learn more about SOS #35: Here are other ways to "wake up" your Mission element. If you're feeling sluggish, you can pump up your internal fire and get your energy moving with this simple exercise. All you have to do is gently pat your head, face, arms and hands (full length, both front and back), trunk, and then finish with your legs and feet. If you wish, you can do a few rounds and increase the strength of your patting with each round. All told this takes just a few minutes, after which you'll be raring to go.

#36: The 5 Rites of Rejuvenation

Learn more about SOS #36: Widely considered to be one of the greatest anti-aging protocols known, these exercises were first publicized in the West in 1939 by Peter Kelder. In the *Eye of Revelation*, Kelder tells a story of a British intelligence officer who brought this "Fountain of Youth" back with him after he had stayed for years in a Tibetan monastery in the Himalayas. The rites are reputed not only to reduce stress, but also to significantly increase energy, vitality, youth, and positively affect the health of all the systems in the body.

There are many websites that demonstrate the Rites and discuss their efficacy. You can download a free copy of *The Eye of Revelation* at t5t.com/The-Eye-of-Revelation-by-Peter-Kelder-Original-1939-Version (that link is about two-thirds down the landing page). This version of the book has commentary from teachers of the rites. And, this same web site has other services available if you wish to develop the 5 Tibetans practice further.

#37: Set a Strong Intention

Learn more about SOS #37: I was introduced to the Bagha technique from yogic meditation practice and the Tai Chi training of Dr. Chunyi Lin of Spring Forest Qigong. (See Learn more about SOS #6.) Burt Goldman, the "American Monk" also uses the Bagha technique in his work. (You can check out seven free meditation/relaxation lessons from Goldman at "theamericanmonk.com/online/lessons/ meditation-guide".)

The three-finger anchor technique is also used in the Silva Method to lock in images of your intentions for quick recall. (You can check out the Silva Method and get a free Silva Starter Kit by visiting silvamethod.com.)

#38: Just Do It!

Learn more about SOS #38: Sometimes worry, doubt, over-thinking, indecision, and/or procrastination can paralyze you. Maybe you don't feel that you have enough data to make a good choice, but circumstances are forcing you to deliver a decision by end-of-business day. You find yourself in a position where you can't delay a moment longer.

Despite your rising discomfort, it is imperative that you ACT. (Read about pragmatism and the action-learning cycle in Learn more about SOS #28.) In order to reduce stress and solve the problems confronting you, you need to experiment by acting on your environment. This is the only way you can gather relevant feedback, learn and adapt, make course corrections—then act yet again to learn yet more. Action, as Charles Sanders Pierce stated, is necessary for evolution, growth, and survival. Being an armchair philosopher or a Monday morning quarterback will not reduce your stress and it won't get you anywhere near your goals. So…stop sitting there. ACT!

#39: Activate Your Energy (The 20-Second Rule)

Learn more about SOS #39: Read more about activation energy in the classic book *Flow: The Psychology of Optimal Experience* by Mihaly Csikszentmihalyi and the more recent best-selling book *The Happiness Advantage* by Shawn Anchor. (Refer to his chapter on the 20 Second Rule.) You may also want to view Csikszentmihalyi's TedTalk "Flow, the Secret to Happiness" at ted.com.

There's almost no limit to how you can use the 20-second rule to change your life for the better. For example, if you want to stop watching so much TV, hide the remote and put some good books where it used to be. Make sure that wherever you hide the clicker will take more than 20 seconds (and some physical labor) before you'd be able to put your hands on it.

And if you want to exercise first thing in the morning, put your clothes in the path you take between your bed and the front door. If that doesn't work and your mate doesn't object, sleep in them until your new morning exercise habit is firmly in place. You may also want to place your alarm clock across the room so you're moving before you even know it.

By activating your energy, you're taking strong steps to achieve your goals and integrate healthier habits into your life.

#40: Dance, Stomp, Drum

Learn more about SOS #40: Be brave! Claim your light-on-your-feet self, the one who can move and sway and have a GREAT time, even if it's just for a few moments on your work breaks. And if you're a really adventuresome spirit, you can take a page from Studs Terkel's classic *Working.* In this famous book, Terkel described a San Francisco bridge toll taker who would dance between handing out tickets. Drivers would get in his line just to enjoy the party. Dancing may not be possible in your work, but it's worth thinking about. For example, David Hennessy, one of my former colleagues, and I would do a happy dance in the halls [out of sight of clients] whenever he landed a new contract. It still makes me smile to think of those breakout celebratory moments.

Here are some videos of dancing workers for you to enjoy: first is (v=BMnUu0IskaQ&list=SP51A3D1CEAF24256C&index=2), a traffic cop; the second is a phenomenal street performer (v=zWEqkJ4iw7A) who certainly is marching to his own beat.

As you can see from the above videos, you don't have to take lessons to learn how to dance, stomp or drum—you can just find your own rhythm and move accordingly. However if you want to improve your moves, you can check out lessons of every possible kind on YouTube. Here are some instructional references to get you started:

- salsa dancing (v=PfDVnX4j3-w)

- belly dancing; (v=KBqXxXL-6jo)

- hip hop; (v=q2s6tCn2y6Y)

- stomp dance sample (v=fwaYnJ2ogQk) and instructions (feature=player_detailpage&v=ngvyIZb2uQ8)

- drumming using household items (feature=player_detailpage&v=0OUEUyelo5Y)

And if you like any of these, you can take lessons in real-time, real-life with your mate or a very good friend.

#41: Stand Up

Learn more about SOS #41: If you're working at a desk for long hours, you are more like to suffer from back problems and gain weight. Sitting overly long can also contribute to mental sluggishness, tiredness, diabetes, and higher cholesterol. It is now thought that serious illnesses, such as cancers and heart disease, are linked to our general inactivity—so much so that a new catch-phase has been coined: "sitting is the new smoking".

Here's a statistic that may surprise you: most of us sit for 9+ hours per day (which is much more than we sleep)! But there's some good news on the horizon. A recent workplace study found that people who sit *even one hour less per day* reported feeling significantly more happy and healthy. And if that's not motivation enough, remember that you'll burn many more calories if you stand rather than sit. To further stimulate your thinking on this topic, I suggest doing a web search for "standing desk". You'll come up with many options to create or buy your own standing-desk or a less-expensive standing computer stand.

Another great "Stand Up" idea that's gaining traction is walk-n-talk meetings. My Dutch colleague Auke van Keulen first introduced me to the idea of moving meetings many years ago. He had developed the habit of walking in the nearby woods as part of his executive coaching sessions. This practice has become an integral part our work together; it is a wonderful way to refresh and restart our conversations because we always return with exciting ideas. My experience is that moving meetings are a civilized approach to work (not to mention, a great way to exercise). I have held such meetings with some of my adventuresome clients; it seems particularly helpful to break up blockages when they are stuck. Happily, the walk-and-meet idea is spreading. (See ted.com/talks/nilofer_Merchant_got_a_meeting_take_a_walk or fastcompany.com/3007078/best-meetings-happen-around-block.)

#42: Short Bursts

Learn more about SOS #42: Early studies comparing short burst exercisers versus regular exercisers show considerable promise: that is, both test groups had similar increases in oxygen capacity, reductions in blood sugar, and sustained weight loss. Moreover, proponents of short burst workouts contend that this is a better approach for longevity. You will need to try it out for yourself to see what you think.

Caution: If you are in poor health, it would NOT be wise to leap right into this. Use your head; talk to your doctor; perhaps you'll need to get into better shape before trying short burst exercise.

Check out the following information about short burst workouts:

- dailymail.co.uk/health/article-2255867/Is-minutes-week-exercise-need-fit-Scientists-say-ideal-fitness-regime-involves-intense-bursts-activity.html

- nhs.uk/news/2013/06June/Pages/Are-short-intense-exercise-bursts-enough-to-stay-fit.aspx

- the science behind this movement (v=I4rl50IIPx0)

- longevity and fat loss (v=TF2oPum60sQ)

#43: Do One Thing

Learn more about SOS #43: Scientists have used MRIs to study the brain's response to handling multiple tasks. Apparently multi-tasking creates a "response selection bottleneck" where the brain is forced to respond to several stimuli at once. As a result, people do "task-switching"— i.e., they focus on one thing, and then on the next. Unfortunately, task-switching results in time *lost* because the brain has to determine repeatedly which task to perform in a given moment.

This "adaptive executive control" determines the priority and order of tasks to be addressed (*again, one at a time*).

Unfortunately, we experience unintended consequences when we attempt to manage overwhelm by multi-tasking. This includes increase in stress hormones, loss of memory, dissatisfaction, impatience/short-temperedness, attention disorders from constant stimulation, decreased ability to tolerate silence, and disinterest in spending time with others. (Not to mention, reducing our oxygen capacity because we are barely breathing as we try to do the impossible!)

If you're still not convinced, here's a brilliant article by Christine Rosen (http://faculty.winthrop.edu/hinera/CRTW-Spring_2011/TheMythofMultitasking_Rosen.pdf), plus some evidence that even the business community is starting to see the error of its ways (http://business.time.com/2013/04/17/dont-multitask-your-brain-will-thank-you/ and "The Truth about Multi-tasking" at entrepreneur.com/article/224943.)

#44: Shake it, Baby, Shake it!

Learn more about SOS #44: This quick workout loosens tight muscles, increases flexibility, brings oxygen into your whole body, and gets your blood pumping. It also releases built-up toxins and blasts you into a cleared-out mind. Interestingly, even fidgeting (small intermittent shaking like finger tapping, leg shaking, or simply moving around) can burn 350 extra calories a day! (No wonder those fidgety types are often thin.)

You can also "shake it" by doing the hokey pokey (one of the early shake-it practices) along with these YouTube videos:

- Cartoon hokey-pokey (v=UDmCSvqhhol)

- Hip-hop hokey pokey (v=Jpym9B0ype4)

You can also check out SOS #40—dance, stomp, drum—for other great ways to "shake it".

All of the above suggestions are low-tech ways to vibrate your body. Some people claim that whole-body vibration can help you lose weight—and there are now machines designed to help. You can check out the pro and con thinking on the topic of whole-body vibration by reading the following articles:

- livestrong.com/article/401694-does-vigorously-shaking-your-body-make-you-lose-weight/

- mayoclinic.org/healthy-living/fitness/expert-answers/whole-body-vibration/faq-20057958

#45: Make a Decision: Change, Accept or Leave

Learn more about SOS #45: These honest decision options should reduce your stress. What does NOT work well—and only increases your stress and everyone else's—is to complain or be silently resentful while still taking no action. Such a passive-aggressive response causes you to lose power, confidence and self-respect the longer you stay stuck in this embattled no-man's land.

We know change is hard, but there are ways it can be done more easily. (Look to *The Balancing Act's* CHANGE process in Appendix A.) You can also check out Alan Deutschman's excellent book *Change or Die*.

#46: Never Fail

Learn more about SOS #46: Go to pstec.org to learn more about Tim Phizackerley's proprietary methods and the many exciting programs he has built.

Phizackerley's has been getting remarkable results with this work, and he is building a worldwide community of practitioners. (Go to Learn more about SOS #54.)

#47: Reduce Resistance

Learn more about SOS #47: If your resistance is keeping you from doing something you genuinely need or want to do, it is vital to reduce it. To start, you can refer to SOS #39 (the 20-second rule) as a practical way to reduce internal resistance.

HOWEVER, it is important to first determine what you do and do not want to do, i.e., to protect your boundaries so you can be sure that you, and no one else, is setting your priorities.

It is a vital part of the Mission element that you know your own agenda and respect your desires. For example, if you're in a tug-of-war with a colleague about whose duty it is to write a report, or with a family member about whose turn it is to vacuum the carpet, it's likely that BOTH of you are experiencing resistance. What you need to do is listen to your internal resistance so it can school you about what is the most appropriate action. That way you're less likely to take advantage of others, and they are less able to take advantage of you. The Mission element helps you strike a good balance in these daily issues: i.e., it forbids you from becoming a doormat while also providing you with the energy you need to happily do your share of the work.

#48: Power Poses

Learn more about SOS #48: Amy Cuddy, a social psychologist from Harvard and her research partner, Dana Carney of Berkeley, have studied power dominance behaviors in primates. It is from their research results that the concept of power poses has been popularized.

I think the most remarkable thing about Cuddy and Carney's research is the data demonstrating how much the poses positively affect body chemistry within a mere *two minutes!*

For example, pre and post saliva tests bracketing those two minutes show increases in testosterone (+8%) and decreases in the stress hormone cortisol (-25%) for high-power posers.

In sharp contrast, those poor control subjects who were asked to hold low-power poses for two minutes had negative effects (a decrease in testosterone [-10%] and worse yet, an increase in the stress hormone cortisol [+15%]).

So…sit up straight! There. That's better. Become a power-poser and let the rest of the world see the real you. Use this breakthrough research to simultaneously reduce your stress and increase your sense of personal and professional power.

#49: Choose Your Weapon (Conflict Style)

Learn more about SOS #49: Take the Thomas Hartman Conflict Management quiz so you can discover your preferred conflict style. (Go to ncsu.edu/grad/preparing-future-leaders/docs/conflict-management-styles-quiz.pdf.)

Notice that you may use different conflict styles with certain people or situations. Because each "weapon" has distinct advantages, you would be wise to avail yourself of all of these ways of handling conflict. By observing yourself in action while you practice these, you can more intelligently decide what style will work best in which situations.

#50: Now Power

Learn more about SOS #50: You can learn more about this and similar techniques by reading Eckhart Tolle's books, *The Power of Now or The New Earth*, or by visiting eckharttolle.com. Check out this excellent site, where Tolle shares many free resources, including a self-directed course, videos and articles.

#51: Respect Your Desires

Learn more about SOS #51: Worthy desires have the potential to call us to greatness, whereas ignoring what we desire can cause us to deny our native impulses and to contract, becoming a smaller, less successful person.

The underlying issues in dealing with our desires are sufficiency and purpose. Unchecked desire that is not tethered to our real needs becomes insatiable appetite or consumerism, whereas ignoring life-affirming desires dampens the fire inside us and keeps us from experiencing life's many joys.

To learn more about the importance of having a *burning desire*, read the classic works of New Thought leaders such as Wallace Wattles and Napoleon Hill, whose challenging landmark works have stood the test of time. YouTube carries several audiobook versions of Napoleon Hill's *Think and Grow Rich* and Wattles' famous 1920 text *The Science of Getting Rich*. Note that although these authors focus on wealth-creation, these principles are to be applied to every burning desire you wish to create in every aspect of your life. Because these are densely written works, I recommend bookmarking them so you can return regularly to contemplate and absorb them in small doses.

Learn More about INTERACTIONS Techniques

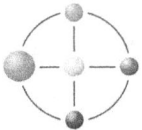

To discover how Interactions can move you from stress to success, please read the Interactions element description that begins SOS Chapter Four, Section I. You can also read the Interactions chapter in *The Balancing Act* (pages 131-142) to see how this element affects your life, relationships and work. (Go to http://balance.thecoreporation.com to read about TBA.)

#52: Experience Compassionate Element of Interactions

Learn more about SOS #52: You can also complete a Relationship Balance Sheet (page 9 of TBA) to start this Interactions section. It might also be helpful to do an *inventory* of your relationships. I've listed below a number of inventory questions to stimulate your contemplation on this matter. The below questions address the health of your *personal* relationships. You can do a similar assessment for your work relationships (colleagues, customers, employees).

- What individuals are most supportive of who you are when you at your best? Who supports your dreams and helps you accomplish your mission?

- Who do you most love, admire and respect? Who cares for you, and who are the people for whom you care?

How intimate, honest, loving and attentive are your relationships? How much time do you spend with the most important people in your life? How do you show love? How do you help each other grow and evolve?

- What good people have passed out of your daily life? Can you reconnect with them? How and when will you do so? What people do you need to forgive—and whose forgiveness do you need to request?

Write these insights in a journal or put into a document you can readily access. The point of such an inventory is to call your attention to relationships you most value, and to encourage you to do whatever is necessary to keep them healthy.

#53: Transform Negative Emotions (EFT)

Learn more about SOS #53: I think of EFT as a self-help combination of acupressure and cognitive behavior therapies. This handy tool has gathered a great deal of attention in the last decade, and is currently undergoing considerable research in many countries. EFT works in part by sending physical and verbal soothing signals to your brain, which in turn dramatically lowers cortisol—by as much as 25% in one study!

And the good results are mounting. For example, there is a 5-year study at John Hopkins where researchers are using EFT for returning soldiers with Post-traumatic Stress Disorder (PTSD). At the three-year mark, this study reported a staggering 63% reduction in trauma symptoms. EFT has also been used successfully with victims in war zones, natural disasters, violent crimes, and mass shootings. So...just think of what it could do to reduce your day-to-day anxiety!

Another benefit of EFT is that it can help you proactively enhance physical and mental performance—so don't restrict its use only to reacting during difficult moments. Here are additional EFT videos and websites for you to explore: "Try it on Everything" (v=9jTNHHTxG40); TappingSolution.com; EFTUniverse.com; tap4health.com/blog/.

In addition to EFT, there are many other ways to transform overwhelming feelings. One popular anger management strategy is to break up things or beat on pillows in a safe room. This is considered a cathartic approach that releases potentially dangerous rage that's built up inside you. Another is to go somewhere you can have an uninterrupted crying jag to release sadness and grief. And lastly, you can simply acknowledge how you feel and let it be just what it is for now. (See Reduce Resistance, SOS #47.)

Caveat: Please take care to not disturb others when doing any of these processes. Most people are uncomfortable with emotional release of any kind, so be certain no one tries to interrupt or "rescue" you.

#54: Percussive Suggestion Technique (PSTEC)

Learn more about SOS #54: PSTEC audio technology builds on psychological principles and recent discoveries from neuroscience to create a unique system that combines positive suggestion with pattern-interruptions of our previously conditioned negative emotional responses. This remarkable tool is now used widely around the world both for self-help and in therapeutic settings. (In a 2011 survey, 90% of therapists, counselors and coaches rated PSTEC "very effective".)

Go to pstec.org where you can read client statements, FAQs, and community forum. The testimonials on the home page practically glow. I encourage you to try it out; it's very easy to follow along to the free PSTEC click tracks.

You may also want to explore any of the PSTEC especially tailored programs to help you tackle specific stress-related problems (such as weight, phobias, PTSD, panic attacks, smoking). PSTEC is designed to remove feelings associated with any unhappy memories of the past or fears about the future. It scrambles the thoughts and feelings associated with prior (or anticipated) bad experiences so they no longer make any sense and it's easy to let them go.

The goal of PSTEC is to delete all debilitating emotions so frightening experiences become smaller in your mind; it's as if PSTEC drains all the color and power out of those feelings and scary images, so they loosen their grip on you. Many of my clients have found PSTEC very useful. For example, I had a client who was afraid he would perform poorly in an important job interview. Together we walked through the PSTEC process during a session. This dramatically reduced his anxiety and stopped him from imagining the worst possible outcomes. As a result, he wound up presenting himself very well.

#55: Tend and Befriend

Learn more about SOS #55: The primary human stress response has been characterized, both physiologically and behaviorally, as "fight-or-flight." Although fight-or-flight may characterize the major physiological responses to stress for both males and females, behaviorally, females' responses are more often marked by a pattern of "tend-and-befriend." *Tending* involves nurturing activities designed to protect the self and offspring; these promote safety and reduce the build up of toxic stress. *Befriending* is the creation and maintenance of social networks that may aid in this process.

The bio-behavioral mechanism that underlies the tend-and-befriend pattern draws on the attachment-caregiving system. Neuroendocrine evidence from animal and human studies suggests that oxytocin, in conjunction with female reproductive hormones and endogenous opioid peptide mechanisms may be at the core of the Tend & Befriend response. This previously unexplored stress regulatory system has many implications for the study (and better management) of stress.

Unfortunately, most people lack tending and befriending survival strategies. In the past three decades the percentage of individuals who consider themselves lonely in the US has risen from 20% to a whopping 40%! The health risks from loneliness are significant: people who feel lonely are more likely to have an impaired immune system, untreated mental health issues, recover more slowly from surgery, and have greater risks of inflammation, heart disease, and premature death.

Note: Social isolation is reduced only by real human contact. No matter how many Facebook friends or Twitter followers you have, you can suffer from social isolation. Tending and Befriending is a low-tech SOS strategy—and an incredibly powerful one. It proves to us that, in very real ways, when you reach out and welcome someone into your life, your social circle, or your neighborhood, you are helping to heal the world.

#56: Get Over Yourself

Learn more about SOS #56: One way to rewrite your life script so you can star as a hero rather than a victim is to follow the lead of Parsifal. In Arthurian legend, Parsifal was the knight of the Round Table who found the treasure (Holy Grail) all the knights were seeking. Parsifal "got over himself" (and got the treasure) by asking the wounded Grail King these two key questions: "What ails you?" and "How can I serve?"

Unfortunately, these questions are not likely to occur to you when you're stressed. This is a shame, because they often point to a way out of your troubles: i.e., you can change to a better course by finding people who need your help and asking about their needs (what you could do for them that would be helpful). By the way, these are two questions I give my clients prior to interviews. It helps them move into a service-mindset rather than fretting about the many ways they could blow the interview.

Two caveats concerning this SOS technique:

1. When you think someone might need your help, remember the following story. When leaders of an indigenous Amazon nation were approached by people who wanted to help them fight invading oil companies, they were told: "If you are here because you want to 'help' us, please leave now. However, if you are here because you know that your destiny is intertwined with ours, then let us begin our work together." I keep this warning top of my mind whenever I work with at-risk youth or ex-prisoners. I firmly believe that our destinies are intertwined; i.e., their success is my success and our fates are interconnected in a myriad of subtle ways. (See also SOS #87.)

2. Sometimes people refuse to look at their own problems and substitute meddling in everybody else's business instead of facing their own demons. This creates a more subtle form of narcissism. If you have even a slight tendency to do this, please skip this particular SOS technique.

Those caveats aside, this is a potent technique to consider. As a great spiritual teacher responded when asked by a grieving seeker how he could ease his almost unbearable pain: "Do something for someone else; it is the greatest medicine."

You can learn even more about a wide variety of ways to become a real hero by reading *Working from your Core*. In it I describe 10 different Core Types, all of which have gifts for you and can be readily called upon as internal advisors so you can remove limitations and become the great person you want to be. These Core Types are: Innocent, Orphan, Seeker, Jester, Caregiver, Warrior, Magician, Ruler, Lover and Sage. You can also go to thecoreporation.com/services/free_services/ core_type_profile to discover your heroic preferences.

#57: Small Acts of Kindness

Learn more about SOS #57: This idea caught fire when writer Ann Herbert called for people to "practice random acts of kindness, and senseless acts of beauty". She wound up starting a worldwide movement that is very much alive today. See BBC News article: bbc.com/news/magazine-24548023.

If you're interested in joining in the fun, go to randomactsofkindness.org to get more ideas for doing this SOS method. There's even a special section on this website with ideas for teaching children how to practice kindness. For even more ideas, go to: oprah.com/spirit/35-Little-Acts-of-Kindness.

And a word of caution in practicing kindness: please refer to the two caveats mentioned in Learn more about SOS #56.

#58: Smile

Learn more about SOS #58: Smiling activates the release of neuropeptides, molecules that allow neurons to communicate whatever you're feeling to the whole body, and let it know whether you are happy, sad, angry, depressed, or excited.

The feel-good neurotransmitters dopamine, endorphins and serotonin are all released when a smile flashes across your face. This not only relaxes your body, but it can lower your heart rate and blood pressure. Moreover, endorphins are a natural pain reliever and serotonin serves as an anti-depressant. All this contributes to longevity. And, here's the icing on the cake: there's extensive research confirming that others consider smiling people to be more attractive, reliable, relaxed and sincere.

Leo Widrich wrote a terrific article on smiling, including three recommended steps for becoming a better smiler. (http://blog.bufferapp.com/the-science-of-smiling-a-guide-to-humans-most-powerful-gesture). And, here are some real treats guaranteed to make you smile. See film footage from Charlie Chaplin's 1936 film, Modern Times, for which he wrote the classic song "Smile":

- Michael Jackson singing (v=iu-rLA4POkI)

- Nat King Cole (v=5rkNBH5fbMk)

- Judy Garland (v=GAQfwpEDdOw).

And to put an extra smile on your face, here are the lyrics so you can sing along. (Smiling AND singing, what a great idea!)

Smile, though your heart is aching.

Smile, even though it's breaking.

When there are clouds in the sky, you'll get by

If you smile through your fear and sorrow.

Smile and maybe tomorrow

You'll see the sun come shining through, for you.

Light up your face with gladness.

Hide every trace of sadness.

Although a tear may be ever so near,

That's the time you must keep on trying.

Smile, what's the use of crying?

You'll find that life is still worthwhile…if you just smile.

#59: Smile at Three Extra People Today

Learn more about SOS #59: Research has found that seeing a smiling face activates the orbitofrontal cortex, the region in the brain that process sensory rewards. So, when people view a person smiling, they actually feel rewarded. (See Learn more about SOS #58 to understand the many benefits of smiling.)

Smiling is contagious. The part of your brain responsible for the facial expression of smiling resides in the cingulate cortex, an unconscious automatic response area. In one European study, subjects were shown pictures of several emotions: joy, anger, fear and surprise. When the picture of someone smiling was presented, the researchers asked the subjects to frown. Instead, they found that the subjects imitated what they saw. It took a strong conscious effort to turn that smile upside down. So when you smile, most people can't help but smile back.

In *The Happiness Advantage*, Shawn Anchor talks about "mirror neurons" (specialized brain cells that mimic the feelings and actions of the people around us). In his now-famous smile experiment, Anchor pairs up participants. Person B's assignment is to do ANYTHING BUT smile while Person A is smiling at them. Within a minute or two, more than 80% of pairs are laughing out loud at their failed efforts to keep from smiling. This "mirror" phenomenon goes a long way to describing the reasons for the (positive or negative) emotional contagion we experience every day. It also is a strong argument for smiling so as to create an upward emotional spiral at work and home.

#60: Try Laughter Yoga

Learn more about SOS #60: This relatively new stress-busting technique combines a) laughter, with b) deep breathing yoga techniques, and c) the support and emotional contagion of community. Much as the body and brain cannot differentiate between real and fake smiling, they also cannot differentiate between real and fake laughter. Even a few minutes of Laughter Yoga will provide stress relief (more oxygen to your brain, heart and body). Check out Kataria's TedTalk and the Laughter Yoga site to learn several activities that take only a few minutes each. These can easily be used as revitalizing breaks in your day.

Moreover, if you decide to make Laughter Yoga a regular practice, you will produce significant biochemical changes throughout your body that reduce stress hormones, improve blood flow, stabilize blood pressure, reduce pain, improve emotional health, strengthen your immune system—and even increase work effectiveness. All this happens in as little as 10 minutes of sustained "body" laughter.

You can easily sample laughter yoga on your own—and, if you enjoy it, I urge you to find a laughter club or laughter buddies in your area. Laughter clubs provide a safe environment where you can fully enjoy laughing out loud. You won't feel quite so silly—and you'll be less likely to be carted off by the local police. Kataria suggests that, even though you may not feel like laughing, you should "fake it until you make it" because the physical, psychological, and social rewards are so significant.

Interestingly, Kataria launched this movement after reading a book that greatly influenced me when I was the CEO of Central Minnesota Group Health Plan: *Anatomy of an Illness* by Norman Cousins. Cousins created quite a stir when he reportedly cured himself of a fatal disease using laughter as his chosen medicine. Read back-story on the Cousins-Kataria link (canada.com/victoriatimescolonist/news/story.html?id=9ad3739 1-0043-4a76-9000-7db7beb40744).

For more information, here is another excellent article (wikihow.com/Do-Laughter-Yoga) and a video of 40 Laughter Yoga techniques (feature=player_detailpage&v=foCQnR39lvl). You can also go to SOS #20 to read more about the health benefits of laughter.

#61: Find a Choir to Join

Learn more about SOS #61: It appears that when you add community to singing, the positive effects multiply greatly. An Australian 2008 study revealed that choral singers rated their satisfaction with life higher than the public—even when the actual problems faced by those singers were more substantial.

A 1998 study found that after nursing-home residents took part in a month long group-singing program, they experienced significant decreases in both anxiety and depression levels. Another study of 600+ British choral singers found that singing played a central role in their psychological health. Research published in the *Journal of Music Therapy* (2004) demonstrated that group singing helped people cope better with chronic pain. And, in many senior centers the power of group singing as a memory trigger is being studied; indicators are that it slows down mental decline and builds self-esteem.

I recommend that you talk to people in area choirs so you can get a sense of their happiness. Go to a concert and see how much you enjoy it. I have been the member of many choirs and can enthusiastically recommend the experience as a terrific stress reliever and happiness-generator. These days I regularly attend concerts by Boston area professional choirs to hear the master classical works. And for just-plain-fun, I have to say that Boston's Mystic Chorale's sing-a-long concerts raise the roof and leave you dancing down the streets.

#62: Loving Kindness

Learn more about SOS #62: The roots of "loving kindness" are deep in multiple religious, where this practice is used to develop the mental habit of selfless or altruistic love. Loving-kindness can create positive attitudinal changes; it acts almost like self-psychotherapy to free your mind from pain, confusion, anger, and hatred towards people who've wronged you in some way. Loving-kindness has the immediate benefit of sweetening and changing old habituated negative patterns of mind.

"Loving-kindness" is an English translation for the Hebrew word "חסד (chesed)". This term is used often in the book of Psalms (1:2), and refers to acts of kindness that are motivated by love. It is said that: "The world stands on three things: Torah, the service of G-d, and deeds of loving-kindness."

Here is a loving kindness meditation video (v=sz7cpV7ERsM) with excellent instructions. And if you wish to learn more, check out the book *Loving Kindness* by Sharon Salzburg.

#63: Green—Yellow—Red Light

Learn more about SOS #63: This technique helps you access feelings so you can make an intuitive-based decision about the safety of your interactions. Use it to decide whether or not you'll spend time with a neighbor or colleague. It also is a great tool to teach children as a protection against predators (who tend to be highly skilled at confusing others' instincts). Many survivors report that something in the back of their minds told them not to proceed despite this nice-sounding-person's urgings. I've heard the same thing from many executive clients who said that "something inside" told them to not take a job that looked so good on the surface. I've found this technique to be very useful for distinguishing between good and bad potential bosses/colleagues/workplace cultures for my clients.

This technique appears simple, but can have far-ranging positive ripple effects. I once had a client whose mother was straight out of "Mommy, Dearest". Consequently her ability to differentiate between good and not-so-good people was a severely under-developed skill. We began playing this Green-Yellow-Red light game to protect her from manipulative people who called themselves her friends. It wasn't long before she became quite astute at picking up emotional signals that told her which people were good news, bad news, or yet-to-be-determined. I was SO proud of the mastery she gained to correctly read people and navigate a smoother road through both her personal and professional lives.

#64: Give (and Get) a Hug

Learn more about SOS #64: Hugging is extremely effective at healing sickness, disease, loneliness, depression, anxiety and stress. Research shows that a deep hug, where two people's hearts are pressed together, provides many health benefits. (See the comprehensive list compiled by Australian yoga instructor, Marus Julian Felicetti at mindbodygreen.com/0-5756/10-Reasons-Why-We-Need-at-Least-8-Hugs-a-Day.html.)

Among these good reasons to give and get a hug are: building trust; feeling connection and a sense of safety; boosting oxytocin and serotonin; and, strengthening the immune system, thymus gland, and nervous system.

#65: Say Thank You

Learn more about SOS #65: Here are some valuable tips to help you graciously give and receive thank yous.

1. Keep your thank you short and sweet so it's easy to say or write. (I use an e-card program that people love; and one of my clients, an investment SVP, sends hand-written thank you cards that they make him stand out.)

2. Find small things for which you can say thank you—and then thank people early and often.

3. If someone thanks you, accept those thanks graciously. (And if you find that difficult, take a moment to consider why receiving gratitude makes you uncomfortable.)

4. If you forget to send a thank you note right away, just do it now (and without emphasizing apologies).

Because this activity is a person-to-person form of expressing gratitude, you will receive many of gratitude's health benefits. Go to Learn more about SOS #89 to see what these are.

#66: Reversal Tapping

Learn more about SOS #66: This is a variation on Emotional Freedom Technique (see SOS #53). It is called "reversal" tapping because it inverts the way the EFT statement is typically made. I have found Reversal Tapping very useful when I need a really fast break-up of emotional overload and didn't have enough time even for a few EFT rounds.

This process has also been useful when I couldn't retreat to a quiet place to do EFT. I've discovered that reversal tapping can be done rather inconspicuously, for example while walking or with hands under the table at a meeting (as long as you take care to keep your arms and upper body still while doing this.)

I learned this technique from the *Crack Your Egg* course by Henk Schram. For more information about this excellent program, go to http://crackyoureggprogram.com/.

#67: Connect with a Critter

Learn more about SOS #67: Numerous studies indicate that connecting with animals goes a long way to "humanizing" us. My sister Dorothy is a truly great biology teacher. I will never forget how impressed I was when she transformed the dynamics of gang rivalry in her Uvalde, Texas classroom. She assigned these at-risk youth specific responsibilities for care and feeding of several class animals. Apparently the needs of their pets resulted in reluctant inter-gang cooperation, and eventually a dramatic improvement in classroom behavior and learning. (I keep telling her that the United Nations needs her!)

Cuddling with other of god's creatures makes us happier and is great for our health. Studies indicate that contact with animals speeds recovery rate for heart attack victims; reduces blood pressure and heart rate; improves therapeutic results for anxiety, mood disorders, marriage counseling; soothes trauma victims (e.g., horse riding as therapy); and it also elevates mood, health and community interaction for nursing home residents. This SOS activity can turn you into a *biophile* (one who loves life and all living creatures).

#68: What Are You Feeling?

Learn more about SOS #68: People can recognize an emotion in less than six seconds. If it's a stress-increasing toxic emotion, you have about 10 seconds to reverse these signals. This is important because at the 16-second-from-trigger mark, your brain will begin flooding your system with stress hormones. The quicker you can recognize what you're feeling in any given moment, the healthier you're going to be.

It is difficult for most us to pay regular attention to how we feel. And sometimes we'd really rather stay busy or numb so we can ignore pain that is percolating below the surface. Unfortunately, ignoring stressful emotions can be hazardous to your health.

And this low-EQ problem goes way beyond the adverse impact it has on our individual health and wellness. Indeed, it has been argued that what the world suffers from today is "e-motion" sickness: unchecked, underground, unacknowledged toxic emotions that are projected onto other people whom we blame for our troubles. (You only have to listen to world news reports to recognize the strength of this point of view.)

Learn More about SOS STRUCTURE Techniques

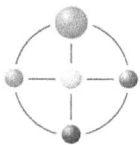

To discover how Structure can move you from stress to success, read the Structure element description that begins SOS Chapter Five, Section I. You can also read the Structure chapter in *The Balancing Act* (pages 165-176) to see how this element affects your life, relationships and work. (To read about TBA, go to http://balance.thecoreporation.com.)

#69: Experience the Steadying Element of Structure

Learn more about SOS #69: This is a good point in the TBA process to do a physical inventory of what is currently working for you and what is not. You can begin by scanning your body for aches, pains, or stiffness. Note any problem areas so you can use the SOS techniques in this or prior sections to feel better. Structure also includes the physical scaffolding of your life, so your inventory can assess structural issues such as: making a budget so you can more carefully monitor your expenses and income, increasing the functionality and health of your living and working spaces, and improving the quality and value of your work products or services.

And lastly, Structure requires that you implement functional processes/habits that will support you in achieving your goals.

This includes having feedback systems in place so you stay in constant touch with your changing environment. This pragmatic feedback keeps you alert so you know when to make course corrections rather than continuing to work inefficiently (i.e., repeating old behaviors and expecting different results).

#70: Show Me the Money

Learn more about SOS #70: There are a many books and programs that address the root causes of money problems. One recent one is *Tapping into Wealth* by Margaret Lynch (in which she helps readers remove emotional and mental blocks to five different kinds of money). It is vital that we solve our money problems in a lasting way, at their roots, because money causes so much distress for so many people. And, although physical paper or coins are just symbols of value, agreed-up social constructs, we need to take every opportunity to reduce the very real distress, pain, relationship problems, and even illnesses that are caused by money concerns.

There are many unfortunate outcomes of our current global monetary system. This first is its staggering inequality (34% of the world's population live on $2 per day or less); many more live without adequate water, food, shelter, and health care. Additionally, too many people define their "value" in terms of how much money they have, others feel desperate enough to do just about anything to get more money—and we have no shared way to define value for truly priceless things such as health, freedom, happiness, love, community, or life itself.

I'm guessing that people who are willing to "do anything for money" are NOT reading this book. (It's unlikely to be making the rounds of political tyrants, unethical business leaders, drug lords, gang leaders, or slave traders—no matter how stressed they are!) However, to a much lesser degree, any one of us can become a slave to money (for example, if we stay in a job that doesn't suit us, just to pay the bills). This is a common way people can forfeit their health, precious time with loved ones, use of native gifts, freedom, or even souls if they're not careful.

The good news is that you can leverage the wealth inherent in each Element of Success to show yourself more money:

1. Core – Get a better job with improved self-esteem, happiness, and awareness of native gifts to leverage.

2. Mind – Be more innovative and cash in on these new ideas; reframe current thinking so creative more often.

3. Will – Increase energy and motivation to accomplish goals; take initiative to land sale or negotiate salary.

4. Emotions – Create healthy connections and network; find people who can help; stay emotionally stable.

5. Body - Carefully manage money; maintain health so can keep working; produce high-value products & services.

6. Source – Leverage connections; understand context so improve value of products/services; increase good luck.

#71: Hydrate Your Body

Learn more about SOS #71: Our bodies are, on average, 60% water (as infants, our bodies are 75% water, but this percentage decreases as we age). In the hierarchy of needs to sustain life, water is second only to oxygen.

Unfortunately, when we get stressed, the body dehydrates in its attempts to deal with that stress (e.g., our muscles tighten, our throats get dry). Sometimes stress signals are misinterpreted as hunger pangs. (Read that again if you tend to do stress eating.) Often, all your body needs is a long, tall, cool glass of water to feel full, rebalanced, refreshed and ready to go again.

#72: Bless What You Eat and Drink

Learn more about SOS #72: There are good reasons why this practice is found across all cultures and throughout recorded history. When you bless your food before eating, it slows you down and allows for conscious eating. When you eat slowly you can actually taste your food. You also can take time for conversation with your family or friends.

Blessing food before eating it tends to make you more grateful for that food. In turn, this slowing down of your mind and body allows both of them to do a better job of digestion and assimilating nutrients. That is, you will eat less and enjoy it more, plus you'll get more value out of it (literally).

Blessing what you eat and drink may have an even more far-reaching impact. There is controversial, but intriguing, research by Dr. Masaru Emoto of Japan, who demonstrated that positive human emotions of love and gratitude can actually change water crystals into beautiful symmetrical patterns and purify it. All you have to do is say is: "Thank you, I love you."

Interestingly, Emoto discovered that the reverse is also true, i.e., negative emotions such as anger or fear will make water molecules misshapen and ugly. So, when you next take a bite of food or drink a glass of water, *bless it rather than stress it*! This practice seems even more reasonable when we consider that nutritious food and clean water are precious global resources. A little appreciation would not be misplaced.

In fact, only a small percentage of the Earth's fresh water is currently healthy to drink (and only 2.5% of the Earth's water is fresh vs. sea water). As a result, drinkable water is now—literally—more valuable than gold (see comparative S&P Water vs. Gold indices as proof). This has caused political and military leaders to discuss how to avoid an international water supply crisis and the eruption of "water wars", particularly in already struggling countries. Happily there are some recent remarkable inventions that make unsafe water drinkable; understandably, these are gaining attention and major investment. (See *HaloSource* as an example.)

To learn more about how blessing your water and food might physically affect you in positive ways, read about Emoto's research at masaru-emoto.net/english and watch this video about Emoto's experiments (v=tAvzsjcBtx8).

#73: Ear Massage

Learn more about SOS #73: Massaging your ear is called "auriculotherapy", i.e., reflexology of the ear. The auricle of the ear (the external, protruding portion) is viewed in some healing traditions as a microsystem that reflects the entire body. According to Western science, massaging your ears reduces stress, increases relaxation, boosts the immune system, and makes you happier by triggering the release of brain endorphins. The Chinese healing systems of acupressure and acupuncture have used ear reflexology for thousands of years to address a myriad of health issues. These health practitioners believe that when you rub, pull, gently twist, or unroll your ears, you stimulate numerous energy points that run through the ears and then into your body.

Here is an instructional video that demonstrates how to do a full ear massage (v=E9x5xKUsYGI). Try it out. It feels great!

#74: Red Flag!

Learn more about SOS #74: If you ignore your body's red alerts, it could have very bad results, indeed—comparable to ignoring red lights on your car dashboard before a major engine malfunction. When your body is screaming at you about the stress and pain it's currently enduring, you are already well on your way to much bigger problems.

So pay close attention to any physical warning signs. Everyone reacts to stress differently, and each body sends out a different set of signals. Some people may not even feel the physical or emotional warning signs until after hours of stressful activities. But when you do notice a stiff back or hear yourself snapping at your friends, listen to what your body is telling you. By noticing how you respond to stress, you can help your body correct itself, reducing the likelihood of complete breakdown.

#75: S-t-r-e-t-c-h

Learn more about SOS #75: Although yoga stretching was considered rather weird only a decade or so ago, it has now become relatively mainstream. Stretching's health benefits include not only reducing stress, but also increasing strength, general fitness, flexibility, and longevity. There is considerable research to support stretching as a complimentary approach for treatment of chronic pain or serious illness. See http://yogahealthfoundation.org/health_benefits_of_yoga_explained; and mayoclinic.org/healthy-living/stress-management/in-depth/yoga/art-20044733.

The word Yoga means *to unite*—but when you're stressed, you're more likely to feel fragmented. Yoga stretching poses were developed as healing practices over millennia, largely in India. They are used to prepare people so they can endure long periods of sitting meditation. Personally, my experience has been that I became "meditative" when twisting into these semi-pretzel shapes because I couldn't concentrate on another thing if I was to keep from falling over. You don't have to be limber benefit from stretching. Just start wherever you are. Listen to your body (don't push it), and then allow these gentle exercises to ease the kinks out of both your body and mind.

Here are some instructions for simple stretching exercises:

- Yoga for beginners (v=Oo0kNeOyH98; 20 minutes)

- Yoga 101 (v=I2yC0Qev_-o30 minutes)

- fitnessmagazine.com/workout/yoga/poses/beginner-yoga-poses/

- http://yoga.about.com/ od/yogasequences/tp/Simple-Yoga-Exercises.htm.

More about the Sun Salutation: This stretching combo is special because it's a holistic series of yoga poses that benefit ALL of the systems in the body, thereby providing you with even more results than individual stretching poses.

The sun salutation is a good way to lose weight and an excellent cardiovascular workout because it stretches and tones all the muscles in the body. I suggest that you use this sequence of yoga stretches not just for stress reduction, but also as a preventive measure to maintain overall good health.

More about Slanting: Moderate inversion decompresses and stretches the spine, allows free flow of blood to the brain, gives you a natural facelift, improves eyesight, increases energy and improves your mood. It also works the cardiovascular system, gently builds a strong core in your body, and helps detoxify the whole system. Check out *Easy Slanting: Relieve Stress in 5 Minutes a Day* by Julia Busch. Busch includes a number of gentle exercises to use while slanting to optimize its effects.

#76: Brain Gym

Learn more about SOS #76: The Brain Gym methodology is taken from the field of Educational Kinesiology. These exercises have been tested for more than twenty years in school settings to improve: overall academic performance, writing, mathematics, reading, spelling, attention and memory. The brain gym website has research archives with articles written by instructors who have used Brain Gym in diverse settings; these reports range from the anecdotal to the statistical to the theoretical.

For more information, go directly to braingym.org. You may also want to jump right in by watching this fun Brain Gym demo (v=VL4an7UC3wA) for children (and adults who like to have fun). You can easily download this video to your smart phone or computer for instant access.

#77: Eat an Apple a Day

Learn more about SOS #77: There is a long list of reasons why eating an apple a day "keeps the doctor away". Because apples are a good source of vitamin C, they decrease blood pressure, improve breathing, and lower blood sugar. Apples also supply vitamin B6 and potassium. Potassium conducts electrolytes that maintain a regular heartbeat and conduct nerve transmissions. Vitamin B6 can reduce stress by promoting the release of the mood-elevating neurotransmitter serotonin—and it is also essential to breaking down fats. Here is a more detailed article: mnn.com/food/ healthy-eating/stories/10-reasons-to-eat-an-apple-a-day.

As it turns out, apples not only promote general relaxation, but also support great sleep. Because they contain a number of sleep-promoting vitamins and minerals, polyphenol antioxidants and almost no fat, they are an excellent option for late-night hunger pangs. Apples even burn fat as you sleep! (How fantastic is that?) See why apples make such a good sleep aide: livestrong.com/article/503595-eating-apples-before-bed/.

#78: Tea Time

Learn more about SOS #78: Tea has been used throughout 5000 years of recorded history in countries across the globe as a medicinal and comforting drink. One reason for the appeal of tea is that it contains antioxidants. (There are large amounts in white and green tea, but black tea has antioxidants also.)

Even today, teas are brewed as medicines in many cultures to treat specific illnesses. I won't use this forum to debate whether or not teas can help cure serious illnesses, nor will I tout the benefits of one tea versus others. However, I do recommend that you do your own experimentation to find the teas you most like. (You'll have hundreds of them from which to choose.)

See the many benefits of tea: doctoroz.com/slideshow/health-benefits-tea; huffingtonpost.com/2012/08/23/tea-health-benefits-cancer-heart-disease_n_1826138.html.

#79: Remind Yourself to Eat Slowly

Learn more about SOS #79: Eating slowly is good for your digestion. It prevents you from over-eating because it takes the brain 15-20 minutes to recognize that the stomach is full. And, by chewing your food more, enzymes in saliva have time to break down the food in your mouth. (This is why food gets digested more fully when you take your time eating.)

Think of it this way: the more chewing you do, the less strain you will have on the rest of your digestive system, the happier your body will be, and the less weight you will gain. (Studies have found that people who eat fast are *three times* more likely to be obese than people who eat slowly.)

And if all that doesn't provide you with enough incentive to slow down, remember that you're also likely to save money on your food bill by eating more intelligently (i.e., slowly).

#80: You Snooze → You Win!

Learn more about SOS #80: Everyone needs a nap now and then, according to the National Sleep Foundation (NSF). Brief naps have many health benefits: they help improve brain function, job performance, alertness, stamina, and mood.

The NSF reported a study from the National Aeronautical Administration (NASA) on sleepy military pilots and astronauts; this research found that naps improved their performance by over 30% and alertness by over 95%! (Note: A 15-20 minute nap is optimal; but grab whatever snooze time you can.) For people who have a long day, a nap can be a lifesaver. I typically get up early and meet with international colleagues or clients both before and after normal work hours, so a mid-day nap makes me feel like a million bucks.

Go to sleepfoundation.org for a list of famous nappers, to read articles about the power of napping, and for tips for making naps even more effective:

- http://lifehacker.com/5950732/the-science-of-the-perfect-nap

- webmd.com/balance/features/the-secret-and-surprising-power-of-naps

- http://voices.yahoo.com/ health-benefits-power-naps-cat-naps-5528437.html.

#81: Treat One of Your 5 Senses

Learn more about SOS #81: When you're feeling stressed, it could be due in some part to sensory overload. This can cause malfunctioning in your perceptual systems, which in turn severely reduces your ability to function effectively.

You can use this SOS tool to stop that overload, i.e., to have your sensory systems work *for* you rather than against you. Paying attention to, and directly soothing, one of the five senses is a simple and powerful way to reverse a potentially downward spiral.

I encourage you to take short "time out" breaks during which you can give yourself a variety of sensory treats. (See SOS #13 for reasons why short breaks are such a good idea.) Find pleasure and enjoy stress relief throughout the day by going directly to, and remedying matters, at the sensory source.

#82: Take a Nature Break

Learn more about SOS #82: Nature quickly connects us to our best internal state. As soon as we breathe in the harmony of our surroundings, we shift the throttle down a notch to a more natural pace. Our blood pressure returns to normal, our thoughts quiet, and our whole system slows down. Moreover, in green tree-lined or sea-breezed natural areas you will find that clean air is in greater supply, and that restorative silence or beautiful nature-sounds abound.

To start, just make a list of nearby parks, nature trails, hiking areas, or arboretums. Locate a park that's off your commute route. See where you can hike, go fishing, or rent kayaks for an outing with the family this coming weekend. Listen to news and weather reports for notices of meteor showers or possible days off to play in the snow or dance in the rain.

(Caveat: Some people—especially citified youth—tempt fate by standing on the sea wall to gage how strong the waves are as a Nor'easter approaches, or refusing to wear unflattering boots when a blizzard is predicted, or climbing to a higher vantage point for a better view of the approaching lightening storm. Please teach them early how best to respect Mother Nature's power while still urging them to enjoy her beauty.)

#83: Schedule Stress Breaks

Learn more about SOS #83: Writing it down will help you remember to take an SOS break. Here's why: when writing with a pen on paper, or typing notes into your computer, you are stimulating a collection of cells in the base of your brain known as the reticular activating system (RAS). The RAS is the filter for all the information your brain needs to process, and it gives more attention to whatever you're currently focusing on.

In other words, the physical act of writing/typing brings the information to the forefront and triggers your brain to pay close attention. In turn, this action increases your odds that this new habit of scheduling will help you keep SOS dates with yourself.

#84: Get a Boost from Brain Food

Learn more about SOS #84: For more information on what brain food is—and is not—look to these articles: webmd.com (search "brain food" for archived articles on research findings); huffingtonpost.com (search "brain food" for *Brain Food: Super Foods to Improve Your Cognitive Function*).

You can also go to bbcgoodfood.com (search "brainpower" for article entitled *10 Foods to Boost Your Brainpower*) and read an excellent article by David DiSalvo: *What Eating Too Much Sugar Does to your Brain* at forbes.com.

#85: Clean-Sort-Move-File

Learn more about SOS #85: Feng Shui is a Chinese spatial relations science that has been developed over 4000 years. This system contains many rules about how best to arrange physical items into a harmonious order that optimizes the healthy flow of energies in rooms, homes and buildings.

Although the principles of Feng Shui are complex (and its efficacy disputed in the West), you can borrow simple advice from this huge body of knowledge—such as beautifying your spaces with flowers, art objects, or colors that lift your spirits.

For more information about how to put this ancient art/science to work for you, go to http://fengshui.about.com.

Learn more about SOS SYNERGY Techniques

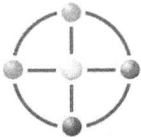

To discover how Synergy can move you from stress to success, read the Synergy description that begins SOS Chapter Six, Section I. You can also read the Synergy chapter in *The Balancing Act* (pages 215-226) to see how this quality that unifies the five Elements of Success can positively affect your life, relationships and work. (To read more about TBA, go to http://balance.thecoreporation.com.)

#86: Experience the Flow and Ease of Synergy

Learn more about SOS #86: Just as you had the option of doing inventories in the two prior chapters, you might benefit from doing an inventory of the many different kinds of systems that support your life and work. These systems can range from the physical infrastructures of your city and nation, the interconnecting environmental web, economic, familial, governmental and political systems. Observe. Make notes.

As you recognize each system that supports your work and life, allow yourself to *feel* your connection to it. Express gratitude silently for all these allow you to accomplish. It is wise to take some time out to contemplate all the systems that make possible everything you do day to day. What's more: it's only by understanding how these systems already support you that you'll be able to leverage them so you can achieve even more.

#87: Ho'oponopono

Learn more about SOS #87: The Hawaiian Shamans believed that Ho'oponopono helps us see and then cure the dark, hidden corners of our own souls. They also believed that when we take responsibility for healing ourselves, we also heal others to whom we are _connected by invisible threads_ (predating physics' "superstring theory" by millennia.)

Ho'oponopono will allow you to transform distress into an opportunity for connection, forgiveness and healing. You can change your own judgment, distaste, dismissal and blaming into a transformative opportunity in which you reflect on how you might have contributed to the root cause of the problem. (For example, I may have voted for a senator who later voted to shut down mental health facilities, which in turn led to that angry man living on the street and yelling at me as I walk by. Or, when I fill up my gas tank, I contribute in a small but tangible way to a myriad of environmental woes and health issues.) Ho'oponopono is meant to help us realize our interconnectedness with, and our contribution to the problem so we experience compassion (versus guilt) and send blessings through these invisible threads to help to heal the world.

So...when I see heinous crimes, corporate greed, or war crimes reported in the news, I remember the phrase "Judge not, lest ye be judged". This theme occurs in major religions and also Jungian psychology, which describes a *shadow nature* that exists inside each one of us. When I use this SOS technique, I acknowledge that, under terrible circumstances, I too could do horrible things. By helping me contemplate my own hidden dark sides, this simple but powerful four-part phrase allows me to heal and integrate the otherwise unacknowledged shadows inside me.

And there's another reason to do this or other forgiveness practices: it's very healthy! Studies show that forgiveness not only reduces blood pressure, depression, anxiety, and the risk of addiction, but also improves mental health and strengthens relationships. What's more, it improves our spiritual health and personal evolution; or as St. Francis advised: "It is in giving that we receive. It is in pardoning that we are pardoned."

See Dr. Ihaleakala Hew Len at miraclesandinspiration.com/hooponopono6.html or read *Zero Limits* by Len and Joe Vitale.

#88: The Healing Code

Learn more about SOS #88: Alexander Lloyd, inventor of the Healing Code, argues that stress is at the root of all illness. Therefore, he says, every time you have a health problem you should ask yourself: "What stress is causing this problem?" and "How can I eliminate it?" Lloyd believes that The Healing Code activates the body's powerful natural healing centers to remove stress and that in turn allows the neuro-immune system to do its job.

It is a complete mystery to me why *The Healing Code* works, but this potent self-help technique now has considerable research to demonstrate its efficacy in healing problems ranging from serious diseases to small maladies to general emotional distress. The proponents of this technique believe that it addresses the "heart" or emotional roots of your current problems. I find it to be extremely calming, and have often used it to reduce my own toxic stress before going to sleep.

Lloyd contends that the root causes of many diseases lie deeply below our conscious mind's ability to access and heal them. He argues that most of us have cell memories, negative images and limiting beliefs from early years that create present-day problems. The Healing Code, then, addresses the invisible root causes of toxic stress and heals them in a gentle way.

To learn more, I recommend Alexander Lloyd's book, *The Healing Code: 6 Minutes to Heal the Source of Your Health, Success, or Relationship Issue,* and also his community website (http://thehealingcodes.com). You can also watch Diane Eble, editor of *The Healing Code* in this demonstration (v=61xy5nlOUOw) &/or visit healingcodescoaching.com. At both of these websites you can access many resources, including samples of "truth statements" to repeat while doing the 6-minute Code. You can experiment with these statements until you find those with which you're most comfortable—and you can also create your own.

Caveat: Sometimes people from other traditions are offended by the overtly Christian approach of the Healing Code and truth statements. However, several of my clients have substituted statements from other traditions and the Healing Code still works wonders for them—e.g., an Islamic or Jewish prayer or a general positive statement such as "I am That, I am".

#89: Express Gratitude

Learn more about SOS #89: When stress hits hard, we tend to focus on what's wrong with our immediate situation. I know that "counting your blessings" at these times seems counterintuitive, perhaps frivolous or even a bit crazy because we are trained to focus on the problem at hand so we can solve it ASAP.

However, a direct approach can sometimes get us stuck further in the mud of the problem rather than helping to get us out of it. Indeed, focusing on our troubles overly long can become like staring into the eyes of the Hydra: we lose perspective; we get paralyzed; we complain; our creativity flees from us—and our difficulties become worse.

Truth is, you've likely gotten so accustomed to the thousands of good things composing the "basso-continuo" of your life that your tendency is to stop noticing everything that's going right for you. Indeed, for most people who are reading this book: you have a roof over your head; you have food to eat and water to drink; your health is generally good; your friends and family enjoy being with you; your heart is beating without your managing it, etc. The practice of gratitude will keep you from becoming the kind of whining character who only notices the good in your life after it's gone.

To learn more about the mental and physical health benefits of gratitude, I recommend these books by Martin Seligman, the founder of Positive Psychology: *Learned Optimism* and *Authentic Happiness*. You can also visit Seligman's website (authentichappiness.sas.upenn.edu/Default.aspx) or watch ted.com/talks/martin_seligman_on_the_state_of_psychology. Another good resource about how gratitude contributes to happiness is *The Happiness Advantage* by Shawn Anchor.

#90: OM Sounding

Learn more about SOS #90: OM (or AUM) is considered by numerous spiritual traditions to be the original "seed sound" of creation. In the Bible, Aum is said to be the "Word of God" that created the whole Universe. Among the Australian aboriginals and Pacific Americans, Creation stories include their gods claiming "I Am" and making everything in the world with this sound. In most sound creation stories, the original substance of the world is "resonance" that filled the primeval abyss, and then slowly over time, evolved into the world as we now know it.

Some people contend that "seed sound" Creation stories correspond to astronomy's "big bang" theory of creation.

AUM is considered by many to be as close as human beings can come to replicating that primordial seed sound. Although AUM sounding is best known within the Hindu and Buddhist traditions, there are those who contend that the "Ah-men" conclusion of Christian, Judaic, Islamic, and ancient Greek prayers are related to this universal sound.

What I have noticed is that, once I get going, this sound reverberates throughout my whole body, as if I am my own sound box. It feels GREAT! And certainly, no stress can exist inside me while this profoundly peaceful sound rearranges my attitude and vibrates all my cells into feeling better too.

Chanting "OM" has many health benefits: it deepens your inhalation and lengthens your exhalation (increasing lung capacity); reduces stress, depression, fatigue, and muscle tension; improves sleep and general relaxation. It also increases concentration, memory, energy and an over-all sense of wellbeing. (Specifically, it is believed by practitioners that the first sound "Ahh" particularly helps the spine, the second sound "oooo" targets the thyroid, and the third sound, "mmm" helps the brain to function better.)

To learn more about the creation stories of other cultures, read *The Balancing Act*, which includes a variety of creation stories that correspond to each one of the Elements of Success.

#91: I Am That I Am

Learn more about SOS #91: In the Bible, "I AM THAT I AM" is famously described as the response God gave when Moses asked His name (Exodus 3:14).

The Hindu tradition considers this to be the natural sound of the body as it breathes out ("Ha") and then breathes in ("Sa"). Other traditions call this natural mantra *So ham.* (Here "*hmmm*" is on the inhalation and "*sa*" is on the exhalation).

Other traditions claim that these natural sounds are actually combined; i.e., every living creature creates *So 'ham* on the inhalation (which means "He am I") and *Ham-sa* on the exhalation (which means "I am He").

As you can see by the universality and many variations of the phrase "I Am That I Am", human beings across the globe have much in common—including what we believe to be the sound of Creation that still resonates in our every breath.

#92: When in Doubt, Pray

Learn more about SOS #92: Clinical studies on the effects of prayer have more than doubled in the past decade. Read about this growing body of research in *The Healing Power of Prayer: The Surprising Connection between Prayer and Your Health* (by Chester Tolson Ph.D., Harold Koenig M.D., and J. Charles), or go to webmd.com (search "Can Prayer Heal?" in archive.)

To get you started on this SOS practice, you can a) simply speak from your heart, b) recall prayers of your childhood, or c) try some of these beautiful prayers from around the world. And let me add a great practice I learned from one of my star students: a recovered heroin-addict/ex-prisoner who turned his life around. This man incorporated several of his regular NA and other prayers into a walking breath practice, stating that it greatly invigorated and provided more "heart" to his prayers.

Serenity prayer: God grant me the serenity to accept the things I cannot change; Courage to change the things I can; and the Wisdom to know the difference.

St. Francis: Lord, make me an instrument of your peace. Where there is hatred, let me sow love; Where there is injury, pardon; Where there is doubt, faith; Where there is despair, hope; Where there is darkness, light; Where there is sadness, joy. O Divine Master, grant that I may not so much seek to be consoled, as to console; to be understood, as to understand; to be loved, as to love. For it is in giving that we receive. It is in pardoning that we are pardoned, and it is in dying that we are born to Eternal Life. Amen.

Buddhist: May you shed the foolishness in myself,transforming me into a conduit of Love.May I protect the helpless and poor. May I be a lamp for those who need your Light. May all find happiness through my actions, and let no one suffer because of me.Whether they love or hate me,whether they hurt or wrong me,may they all obtain happiness and realize Nirvana.

Native American (Navajo): As I walk, as I walk, the Universe is walking with me. In beauty it walks before me; in beauty it walks behind me. In beauty it walks below me; in beauty it walks above me. Beauty is on every side; as I walk, I walk with Beauty. (Repeat prayer, substituting: ...In Peace.... in Love...)

Traditional African prayer song: O all ye big things of the earth, bless ye the Lord—bless ye (mountains, elephants, etc.)...O all ye small things of the earth, bless ye the Lord—bless ye (ants, leaves of grass, etc.). All shall be Amen and Alleluia. We shall rest and we shall see. We shall see and we shall know. We shall know and we shall love, We shall love and we shall praise. Behold our end, which is no end.

Islamic prayer: Praise be to Allah, The Cherisher and Sustainer of the Worlds; Most Gracious, Most Merciful; Master of the Day of Judgment. Thee do we worship, and Thine aid we seek. Show us the straight way: The way of those on whom Thou hast bestowed Thy Grace—Those whose portion is not wrath and who go not astray.

Jewish blessing: May we live to see our world fulfilled, May we be a link to future worlds, and may our hope encompass all the generations yet to be. May our hearts conceive with understanding, may our mouths speak wisdom, and our tongues be stirred with sounds of joy. And our tongues be stirred with sounds of joy.

#93: All is Well

Learn more about SOS #93: Louise Hay is a national treasure. Check out her many books, blog, and website. Her new book is actually entitled *All is Well.* You may also want to listen to the exquisite compositions of Hildegard of Bingen, which are terrific for stress reduction and will make you feel that—absolutely--all IS well. Here is a sample (v= Dehwp_drlyq), and I also recommend the CD of "Vision" which was released to great acclaim in 1994.

#94: Healing Circle

Learn more about SOS #94: Many cultures from around the world have some kind of "healing circle" as one of the primary healing tools of their Shamans. Does it work? I know of no controlled scientific studies verifying its efficacy. However, the fact that this beautiful image and its corresponding practice have survived millennia as healing tools across the globe testifies to the esteem in which they are held.

Perhaps the Healing Circle reminds us of our full humanity— and that we contain the same archetypal elements that make up the entire Universe. Perhaps it calls us back to harmony among these qualities when we're feeling out of balance because we've been ignoring some aspects of our nature and overdoing others. I do not know. What I DO know from using this tool for hundreds of clients and myself, is that the archetypal template of the center and four directions encodes valuable healing information for all human beings.

#95: The 5 Element Mantra

(6 seconds…to as long as you wish)

<u>Learn more about SOS #95:</u> It is believed by many traditions that "Namaḥ Śivaya" has such power that the mere intonation

of these syllables does considerably more than relieve your immediate stress. In fact, these syllables are believed to be inherently sacred sounds that vibrate the body into a perfectly integrated, balanced alignment of all the 5 elements.

This mantra is said to soothe the soul, cut the bonds of the intellect so it can see its own ignorance and so that wisdom can burst forth from within. The 5 Element mantra comes from Shaivism, a form of Hinduism that focuses on Shiva as "All and in all"—the 5-part God (Creator, Preserver, Destroyer, Revealer and Concealer). Shaivism is widespread throughout India, Nepal, Sri Lanka, Malaysia, Singapore, and Indonesia. I learned this beautiful practice while studying the meditative tradition of Siddha Yoga. (See siddha.org.)

#96: Find the Roots of Your Distress

<u>Learn more about SOS #96:</u> Unless you find the roots of what's stressing you, I can guarantee that the problem will

return in one guise or the other. One of my personal heroes, business guru W. Edwards Deming (considered the "father" of the Total Quality Movement) believed that about 85-90% of organizational problems are systemic, and that these will recur despite the best efforts of individuals. Similarly, many of our personal problems are systemic and will repeat unless we deal with them at their origins. (As every gardener knows, weeds will grow back if you've not gotten them out by their roots.)

My intention in writing *SOS: Switch Off Stress* was to give you practical tools that provide momentary "first aid" relief so you can push back accumulating stress. It is my hope that this temporary relief will allow you to come back later to find root causes and determine lasting solutions. The questions in this activity are designed to launch you on this worthwhile inquiry.

#97: Get the Binaural Beat

Learn more about SOS #97: Research overwhelmingly asserts that even a little meditation daily can enhance your life span, reduce heart disease, and increase happiness levels. Binaural meditation audios use "multivariate resonance technology" to ease the brain more quickly into a natural meditative state.

For more information about a wider variety of binaural offerings, go to omharmonics.com. I use these meditations daily and recommend them highly.

For more information about the science of binaural beat patterns, go to: monroeinstitute.org/resources/what-are-binaural-beats. There are many binaural beat options available by surfing the web; one that offers an excellent free sleep track is at http://free-binaural-beats.com.

You can also find "whole brain" meditations that use binaural beats for deep relaxation. Go to LucidQuest.com for a variety of free samples there. And here's a fun whole brain functioning video (v=AO_If2RPVPQ&feature=player_detailpage).

#98: Portable Spa Treatment

Learn more about SOS #98: This technique strings together all the Elements of Success into a holistic, entertaining self-treatment that borrows from healing traditions the world over.

I have had great success with this process in speaking engagements; it is such a pleasure to provide participants with a tangible, immediately useable self-help process. People love it, and it's a treat for me to be able to provide a whole room of stressed-to-the-max people with a fast, delightful "spa" treatment. For more information, read *The Balancing Act*, or visit thecoreporation.com.

#99: This Too Will Pass (The Holographic Universe)

Learn more about SOS #99: Quantum physicist David Bohm and neurophysiologist Karl Pribram independently arrived at holographic models of the universe: that the microcosm and macrocosm reflected each other (or as ancient philosophers stated "As Above, so Below; As Inside, so Outside".)

The Balancing Act borrows from both modern science and ancient wisdom by using the concept of Synergy and the images of sacred geometry to reflect the holographic nature of the world. For example, the TBA image forms a perfect circle, a perfect square, a pyramid (with the center as the pinnacle), and a diamond with the center as a point both *Above* and *Below*.

Moreover, the ancients used these same TBA elements to describe the true nature of human beings, the composition of our universe, and how the Microcosm and Macrocosm reflect each other. Interestingly, the ancients described in metaphor and imagery the Holographic reality now theorized by our era's greatest scientists. According to them, we are composed of the same raw material from which absolutely everything (animate and inanimate) in the Universe has ever been shaped as it passed into and out of "reality".

So stop making yourself small—you are timeless, made from the same stuff as stars! Whatever problems you're having today, when put into such a magnificent perspective, are very small indeed. And they too will pass.

To learn more, read *The Holographic Universe* by Michael Talbot, in which he describes the work of Bohm and Pribram—or read their works directly. You can also see *The Balancing Act's* chapter on Synergy. And, you may want to explore New

Thought leader Wallace Wattles' classic 1920 book, *The Science of Getting Rich*, in which he describes how the Formless moves into Form (implicit to explicit) as a "wonderful becoming". (See YouTube audiobook.) Wattles contended that we should participate in shaping that ongoing creation so we have the lives we really want. Wattles describes the Formless life force in this way: "There is a thinking stuff from which all things are made, and which, in its original state, permeates, penetrates, and fills the interspaces of the universe."

#100: Get a Great Night's Sleep (Top 10 Tricks)

Learn more about SOS #100: Sleep has great restorative powers and is vital for your mental and physical wellbeing. This Top 10 list is designed to make sure you get all the nightly repair time you need. Below are the specifics and rationale for each recommendation. I hope you put one or several of these immediately to work for you.

1. Unplug to relieve stress on your whole nervous system. Some stress experts argue that the best thing you can do to reduce stress is to "unplug" from all your electronic devices. This calms your entire nervous system, which is especially important before trying to sleep. For example, your eyes become overly stimulated by TV and computer screens; this makes it difficult for your brain to slow down neural signals. Bear in mind that the closer it is to bedtime, the worse these effects will be for you. (The exception is meditation or relaxation audios that can ease you into deep sleep.)

2. *Avoid bad news.* TV or Internet news is highly sensationalized. Moreover, your mind has a difficult time differentiating between your personal problems and a crisis you're watching that is happening halfway around the world. Take a break from it to get a good night's sleep. Frankly, you need not worry—all the world's problems will be still there for you to think about tomorrow. So just for tonight, let them go.

3. *Your digestion* is designed so that your body completes a second digestive phase while you sleep. This natural cycle completely cleans out your body. However, if you give in to the munchies (which are likely to start in earnest after 10pm), your body will be overloaded with excess food. Your stomach acid rises to meet the task (resulting in heartburn, acid reflux or worse) and toxins build up (including turning into excess fat).

4. *Spend quiet time with loved one(s).* This is the adult equivalent of having Mom or Dad tuck you in and read you a bedtime story. Obviously, having sex with your partner is a tried-and-true way to forget all your troubles and get a great night's sleep. It's also true that being held in love is soothing at a profoundly deep level. If you don't have a loved one close at hand or s/he is occupied, you can call a dear friend or family member. And make that call to a good, sane person—not a drama king or queen who will agitate rather than soothe you.

5. Prepare for tomorrow. This will go a long way to reducing your anxiety and quieting your mind so it doesn't torture you with looping reminders of everything you have to do upon waking. If you feel prepared, you can just exhale and let the day go. You'll rest much more easily if you know you're ready to go as soon as the morning wake-up call sounds.

6. Parentheses (meditate or contemplate before & after sleep). Meditating in the time before bed is a wonderful way to slow down your mind/body and ease naturally into a sound sleep. You can use the binaural sleep meditation audios to make this transition easier. And here's another delicious technique—take two minutes to review all the good things that happened this day. I've found that this makes me feel great in the moment and helps me slip gently into a deep sleep and good dreams.

What's more, if you pause for two minutes to ease yourself awake in the morning (rather than leap into action or worry), you'll capture more of the benefits of that great night's sleep. Allow yourself to remember dreams &/or receive insights. Take a few slow breaths and notice how comfortable you are at this moment, how warm you are under the covers, how quiet things are, how good your body feels, the softness of the morning light, etc. Let yourself smile as you enjoy these sensations. You'll be in action soon enough, but if you pause slightly, you will create a soft, subtle "parentheses" around your sleep—and its restorative qualities will be significantly augmented.

7. Design your own quiet space and time. You know what does the best job of slowing you down. Read a good book, listen to soothing music, snuggle on the couch with your sweetheart, etc. You can turn this SOS technique into several small habits that pay big dividends via a great night week.

8. Eating a half-apple before bedtime will help you sleep better. (Eat it one to two hours before bedtime; see SOS #77 for research rationale.) There are other schools of thought about what foods work best to ease people into sleep: some argue for a hot cocoa, others for a small amount of protein, others for a small helping of vegetables. I advise you to experiment until you determine what works best for you; the reward will be one great night's sleep after another.

9. Shake out those kinks before falling exhausted into bed if your body is still holding on to the stress of the day. For example, you can do some slow stretches, Tai Chi, yoga, massage, or take a warm bath. I also sometimes drift off to sleep by resting my back &/or neck on a warm herbal heating pad (which releases any vestiges of the day's tensions).

10. Early to bed... As it turns out, Benjamin Franklin was right. All sleep hours are not created equal. Humans get their best sleep between 10pm – 6am. (This is why off-cycle work shifts are so hard on people's health.) Interestingly both Ayurvedic medicine and sleep research agree with Ben that "early to bed and early to rise" reflect the body's natural sleep cycle.

#101: The Balance Beam

Learn more about SOS #101: This is a short form of the Balance Beam. My colleagues and I are in the process of developing an interactive application of the Balancing Beam. We will provide updates on its release date at The Balancing Act Community blog (http://thecoreporation.blogspot.com) and @SharonSeivert.

You can also visit thecoreporation.com and Appendix C to find CORE resources that will directly address chronic stress areas that the Balance Beam points out.

———————————————

SECTION III:

APPENDICES

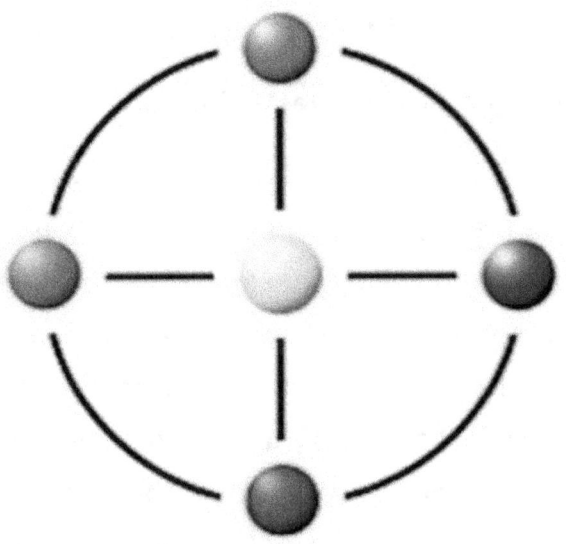

Appendix A. More Background

Appendix B. About the Author

Appendix C. CORE Resources

Appendix D: Synopsis of *The Balancing Act*

APPENDIX A.

MORE BACKGROUND

Sharon's Story:

How I used SOS to meet a Personal Challenge

I began writing *SOS: Switch Off Stress* after my beloved mate, "Matt", had his identity stolen. Although identity theft is a dreadful ordeal for anyone, it is (as I discovered), a much worse trial for immigrants. Matt's social security number was passed around by a group of unsavory characters and used in a number of criminal activities. Because the authorities couldn't figure out who was who, Matt was suddenly under investigation by the US Department of Immigration. After the IRS froze his salary, Matt's employer (himself an immigrant to America) decided to secure an attorney to protect his valuable employee. Unfortunately, Matt was unable to earn a living and his path to citizenship was blocked while the glacially moving investigation wore on for years. This reduction to a one-income family dramatically increased the financial burden on me, and turned our cash flow into a monthly hand-to-mouth endurance contest. Even worse was the constant threat to our relationship during a time when the U.S. government was deporting our foreign-born neighbors in unprecedented numbers.

As the problem continued, I felt as if we were experiencing a real-life version of Kafka's *The Castle*—trapped in a maze by invisible bureaucrats who ranged from the indifferent, to the seemingly callous, to the self-righteous (who assumed they only had to find the smoking gun we were cleverly hiding). I kept telling myself that these people were just doing their jobs, but as the months and years rolled by, my patience wore correspondingly thin.

I mean, really, what were they thinking! As my brother, a senior executive in the National Security Agency once commented: "They're investigating Matt? For the love of God, have they met him? He's about as threatening as a cocker spaniel puppy."

The fact that we were repeatedly given promises that were as-repeatedly broken was disorienting and difficult to endure. Time and again, we were looked in the eye, our hands firmly shaken, and told all was resolved—only to have nothing happen. This required us to start all over with brand new people in a few months. It was maddening.

Also disconcerting was the possibility that I might be considered guilty-by-association and therefore watched as a person of interest. (I do try to be an interesting person). "Mmmmmm…" an Immigration official once commented to Matt: "…and what exactly DOES your girlfriend do when she travels to Holland?" My Dutch colleagues howled when they heard that. However, rather than sink into a state of hopelessness and helplessness, I started to treat the "investigation" in a somewhat flip way: Whenever I heard an unusual click on the phone, I would turn my own paranoia into humor by inviting whoever might be listening to come up to my home office for coffee. Why should anyone wait in a listening station when they could put up their feet here? Besides, I make great coffee!

As time ground on, with a resolution still evading us, I knew I was up against the kind of long term, health-and-sanity-eroding toxic stress that shortens people's lives. I had to do something. So I responded by building my stress management skills even further. Over these years I experimented with all the techniques that wound up landing in this book (and a great many longer techniques as well).

Speaking personally, humor and love became Matt's and my first lines of defense. Many nights we would joke that: "Well, we're much better off than the (Chilean) miners" and "We must be in the years of the skinny cows—after this we'll be in the years of the fat cows..." and "...but we still have our health" and "...thank God we have each other!" and "...how lucky we are to have a roof over our heads."

Counting our many blessings, expressing gratitude in small and large ways, finding things that made us laugh out loud, remaining kind to each other (despite how crabby, exhausted, powerless and out-of-sorts we felt), continuing with our life-purpose work (his art, my writing)—all these steady practices kept us on track and helped us cope with our daily struggles.

I am happy to report that after four years of at-times-crushing problems, we have broken through just as this book is going to press. The attorneys from Matt's sponsor company and a friend from the Justice Department have prevailed upon Immigration to release Matt from any suspicion of wrongdoing—and the Immigration Department has informed the IRS that it's time to "let my people go".

(Can you hear the joyful chorus?)

During these grinding high-stress years, I had ample opportunity to do some serious personal growth and development. Although there were many days when I was profoundly discouraged, most times I opted to choose happiness, pick myself up and take the high road, one small step at a time. Eventually, stress actually became my friend. It taught me some hard truths. It pointed out my weak spots and forced me to deal with them. It compelled me to master new tools that built my chops for surviving, then thriving. As a result, I became more effective and productive than ever; not in a workaholic, reactive, pain-evasive way, but in a steadily proactive, creative, and more balanced way.

Happily, we have lived to tell the tale, and I can now affirm Ralph Waldo Emerson's statement that "What lies behind us and what lies before us are tiny matters compared to what lies within us." Please accept *SOS: Switch Off Stress* as a treasure chest full of the valuable jewels with which Stress, my new and unlikely BFF, rewarded me for taking this internal journey.

SOS: Why You Need to Stop Distress ASAP

SOS: Switch Off Stress is built primarily as a REACTIVE tool, i.e., to help you respond quickly and effectively to the pain of toxic stress. It's vital that you pay attention to SOS distress signals because you need to: a) deal immediately with the challenge that's been brought to your attention, and b) let your system know that "All is well" after you have taken effective action and these stress signals are no longer necessary. This is an intelligent response that respects the design of your body's stress function while simultaneously keeping you from experiencing stress overload (which will happen if stress signals continue unabated).

The techniques in this book are designed to help you stop distress signals as early as possible in the natural alert process, and in this way reduce any chronic damage to your health from this "silent killer". (See the National Geographic's documentary *Stress: Portrait of a Killer*; you can get this landmark film on DVD from National Geographic; it is also available for immediate streaming on Netflix.)

Switch Off Stress respects the brilliant design of your body's interlocking physical and emotional systems, which have evolved over millennia to protect you. (*Saber-toothed tiger approaching from right: Run for your life!*) Simultaneously, SOS urges you to recognize that excessive use of this brilliant design has become a major health threat today—and that you would do well to proactively protect yourself and those you love by integrating stress reduction techniques into your life.

Here is why it's vital to stop toxic stress ASAP: Within a second of your brain perceiving a threat, it reacts to save your life. Your nervous system responds by releasing a flood of stress hormones, including adrenaline and cortisol. These hormones rouse the body for emergency action: your heart pounds faster, muscles tighten, blood pressure rises, breath quickens, and senses become sharper. These changes increase strength and stamina, speed reaction time, and enhance your focus—preparing you to either fight or flee from real dangers.

Details of the stress response:

When a threat is perceived, the brain activates the amygdala, which triggers the hypothalamus, which in turn almost-simultaneously sends signals to the pituitary gland (to secrete the hormone ACTH) and the adrenal medulla (to release the neurotransmitter epinephrine).

This entire chain reaction occurs within seconds.

These chemical messengers result in the production of the hormone cortisol, which increases blood pressure, blood sugar, and suppresses the immune system. Energy is boosted when epinephrine binds to liver cells, which then produces glucose.

Additionally, the circulation of cortisol in the body turns fatty acids into energy, which prepares muscles so they are ready for this emergency response. Additionally, adrenaline

---

> (epinephrine) or noradrenaline (norepinephrine), facilitate
> immediate physical reactions.
>
> All this activity is referred to as the "Fight or Flight" Response.
> Once the originating threat is over, the parasympathetic branch
> takes control and begins its work to bring the body back into a
> balanced state.

HOWEVER, these very same survival responses are quietly killing us today due to constant use, stress overload, accumulated stress, and slow stress recovery. The problem is that, over time, all the systems in your body get worn down and illness results. An example is *adrenal fatigue*, which has become increasingly common and can take months or even years for complete recovery. (See *Adrenal Fatigue: The 21st Century Stress Syndrome* by James L. Wilson or visit adrenalfatigue.org to learn more.)

So, here's the conundrum: the perfect life-saving system that our ancestors passed down to us does NOT function well in the face of our modern era's myriad, more subtle daily stressors. ("*You'd better hand in that report in by tomorrow if you want to keep this job.*" Or, "*I can't pay the mortgage on time this month.*" Or, "*Mom, here's my report card…sorry.*" Or, "*I don't love you anymore.*" Or, "*I feel unhappy—I don't know why.*")

Let me repeat: Too much stress is *really* bad for you! In recent decades allopathic (Western) medicine has extensively studied the adverse effects of stress on human health and concluded that distress is a contributing factor to **90%** of all illnesses. Indeed, the number of diseases affected by toxic stress is staggering. They include, but are not limited to, the following:

- Cardiovascular diseases (high blood pressure, heart attack, stroke, TIAs).

- Digestive difficulties (appetite, weight, irritable bowel).

- Nervous system problems (migraines, psychoneurosis).

- Autoimmune diseases (hyperthyroidism, diabetes, allergies, fibromyalgia, lupus, MS).

- Addictions (drugs/alcohol/smoking/consumerism/eating).

- Anxiety (PTSD, phobias, panic attacks, OCD).

- Genito/urinary (impotence, menstruation issues).

- Cancers (stress adversely impacts all of them).

- Developmental and learning disorders (ADD, dyslexia, problems with learning and concentration).

And there's even more insult to add to this long list of injuries. Excessive stress also kills our brain cells, ruins our sleep, makes us fat, destroys our attractiveness, and ages us before our time. This "calcification" is not limited to physical problems. Distress also erodes our mental and spiritual health, sense of wellbeing, the health of important relationships, work effectiveness—and contributes to social isolation and violence in our families, communities and the world.

The bottom line is that, if untended toxic stress doesn't kill us outright, it makes us (and everyone around us) miserable. By stealing our potential creativity, vitality and joy, ongoing distress makes us smaller, contracted, and less happy human beings.

The problem I find in my own life and in coaching clients is that it's very easy to ignore stress because, really, it's not likely to cause a heart attack in the next few minutes now, is it? My clients argue: *"How can the stress I'm feeling about this one problem really matter to my overall health?"* Or, *"I'll be better as soon as this situation passes."* Or, *"I don't need to deal with this issue right now, do I? Can't I just wait until next week?"* Or, *"If I ignore this long enough, won't it just go away?"*

The excuses for inaction that I love the most include: *"How do I know this technique is going to work for me?"* Or, *"Frankly, I can't be bothered to take time out now to do this."* Or, *"Can't we come back to this at our next session?"* And my all-time favorite: *"I'm way too frigging stressed right now to learn how to manage stress!"*

The underlying problem is that the effects of ongoing stress accumulate relentlessly over time. Here's an analogy: Stress affects your health almost invisibly, much like tiny grains of sand being washed out to sea. By itself, each grain of sand is not worthy of note. Yet, with each passing storm, with each gust of wind, the grains are one-after-another-after-another swept away. The shore is eroded almost imperceptibly—until the protective barrier is so weakened that your beautiful home collapses "suddenly" into the bay.

Make Stress Your Friend to CHANGE for Good

As I keep insisting, stress CAN be your friend. "Stress" is, in simplest terms, just your internal response to a perceived challenge. Stress becomes an ally when it grabs your attention and directs it to a real problem. An example: The back of your neck is tingling because a mugger is following you; or, you're overusing a muscle and the shooting pain is a signal that you should stop. Both of these are example of "good stress" saying: *Hello! There's a problem here. Pay attention. NOW!*

Good stress is called *eustress*. It helps you get out of a warm bed on a cold morning so you arrive on time at work. Good stress can show you where a real problem or imbalance exists. Eustress helps you pay attention so you can find the root of the problem, deal with it, and evolve to a higher level of functioning. The point of good stress is to help you grow; it makes you uncomfortable enough so you'll move out of a stuck place and start moving in a better direction. It forces you to pay attention so you can survive (which is a very good thing, considering the alternative). AND, if you use *eustress* to find the source of problems, you'll be able to resolve long-standing issues and evolve to a higher state of dynamic balance, i.e., what Ralph Waldo Emerson called "a life well lived."

You turn distress into a friend by attending to repeated signals and making a healthy change. Conversely, you turn stress into an enemy when you ignore the signals it sends you. So, in short: it's up to you. It's that simple—most of the time....

For most readers of this book, it is relatively simple to reduce stress "most of the time". However, reducing stress is not always simple for everyone, nor for any one of us all of the time. Here are major caveats to the "It's that simple" statement.

For example, it is very difficult to manage anxiety when you're coping with a life-threatening injury, or a painful physical or mental illness—although many hospitals, physicians, and therapists are now training patients in stress management techniques that have proven effective in controlling pain and speeding recovery. It is also difficult to stop looping stress signals if you're the victim of domestic abuse, a returning soldier, or a refugee from a war zone, all of whom are likely to be adversely affected by Post-Traumatic Stress Disorder.

Other exceptions include toxic stress whose root causes are systemic, political, cultural, familial, or climate-based. In these circumstances, people may not have a great deal of power to change the situation or respond effectively to the threats they're experiencing. For example, people living in poverty, prison, natural disaster areas, refugee camps and war zones have to deal with body-mind-and-spirit-crushing conditions that are difficult for the rest of us to imagine; these people have far fewer options to effectively relieve the distress they're suffering.

However, my colleagues and I have taught SOS techniques to people in many of these groups, so I know what can happen when individuals do whatever they can, wherever they can, and whenever they can to reduce otherwise-intolerable distress. (History has many examples of how regimes toppled or people survived when they managed to keep their cool.) By making very small changes in the face of profoundly challenging circumstances, these heroes significantly increased their own odds of survival, healing and success (and also that of others).

Clearly, every effort you make to reduce stress is worthwhile because repeated ignoring of stress signals is likely to result in physical illness or mental problems or addictions. Although it's hardly surprising that people choose to "self-medicate" to deaden the pain they're feeling from distress, addictions only cause more toxicity and force distress signals underground—which in turn, contributes to creating even more serious disease. (You've likely noticed that *Switch Off Stress* does NOT include any of these rapid—but far less healthy and effective—responses to stress that a great many people use: lighting a cigarette, pouring a stiff drink, popping a pill, turning on TV, cruising the web, eating more, etc.)

I readily admit that changing ingrained stress-response habits is extremely difficult. *This is true even when that change is vital for survival.* In fact, according to groundbreaking research by

Alan Deutschman, **only 1 in 9 people** will actually make a sustainable lifestyle change—even if they are told that they must *Change or Die* (the title of his excellent book). Deutschman discovered that people do not respond in any lasting way to the 3 "Fs" (Fear, Force or Facts), so change efforts based on those are not going to work well.

However, **better than 90%** of Deutschman's subjects successfully made long-term changes when they followed the three "Rs" (Reframe, Relate, Repeat). My colleagues and I were thrilled to discover Deutschman's work because his three "Rs" are contained within the six steps of *The Balancing Act*'s CHANGE process—and show in part why TBA has been so successful in helping clients make lasting changes in life, relationships and work.

TBA's pragmatic, easy-to-follow change process is noted below. These six steps reflect the 5 Elements of Success and Synergy, which provide a holistic and systemic context for Deutschman's recommended three "R" steps in *Change or Die*.

The Balancing Act's 6-Step CHANGE Model

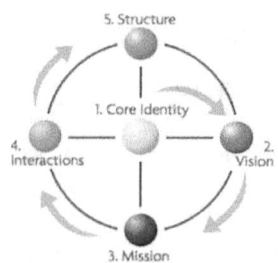

Step 1. Reset (Core): When you recognize things are not working well: stop, pause, and get quiet internally. Don't push yourself to keep going. Instead, become more effective, productive and creative by taking a vital moment to self-reference before starting over. This is a bit like refreshing, restarting or rebooting your computer.

Step 2. Reframe (Vision): Rethink the situation; envision a different future; be inspired with hope; know that change and happiness are possible. Ask pragmatic questions (what is working well, what is not, and why) so you can change the consciousness that created this problem in the first place.

Step 3. Reprioritize (Mission): With this new mental framework, set a strong intention, clarify your priorities, set goals and a clear direction, and then move into action. This revitalization will help you overcome old obstacles as you move decisively into creating the new future you desire.

Step 4. Relate (Interactions): Develop healthy relationships with people who will help you sustain hope, energy, and action. Let go of, or strongly boundary, those relationships that are less healthy and happy for you. Use your emotional GPS to navigate your way and make course corrections.

Step 5. Repeat (Structure): Over time, steadily build more functional habits and skills; keep at it until these changes become your new reality. Implement your learning and new skills by putting them into daily practice so you can grow gradually into all the greatness of which you're capable.

Step 6. Reform (Synergy): When these 5 steps connect, you will have an increased ability to powerfully re-form yourself from the inside out. This is how the change you originally desired becomes thoroughly integrated into your daily life and work until you have a whole new way of being. Because you determined to *reclaim* your personal power and responsibility, you will experience a steady **evolution** that generates more **energy**, a greater experience of **ease**, and perhaps even a positive revolution (*miracle*) in your life.

TBA's CHANGE process is an ongoing dance in which you make constant adjustments in response to the many challenges that life throws your way. This process is designed for you to learn, adjust and adapt to changing circumstances. As a result, TBA stimulates your intuition and creative problem-solving capabilities, improves your resilience, and increases your excitement as you achieve more and more of your goals. Furthermore, TBA's incremental growth process of balancing and counterbalancing allows you to turn insights and small successes over time into a growing conviction that you have everything you need to realize your objectives.

The TBA Change process contains not only Deutschman's three "Rs", but also the classic four-part PDCA and Action-Learning cycles of total quality improvement. By adding the central Core element at the beginning of these four steps and Synergy at the end, TBA turns this *cycle* into an *upward spiral*, i.e., (Be) → Plan/Think → Do/Act → Check/Reflect →

Implement/Have → (Transform). You can remember *TBA's* CHANGE process with the following phrases or key words that reflect these natural evolutionary steps:

CHANGE...

Comes from <u>C</u>entering in your **Core**

Holds all your <u>H</u>opes and your choice to be **Happy**

<u>A</u>lways moves you into <u>A</u>ction

<u>N</u>avigates the way to success via your emotional GPS

<u>G</u>rows you **Gradually** into a person capable of **Greater**...

Ease, Energy, and ongoing <u>E</u>volution.

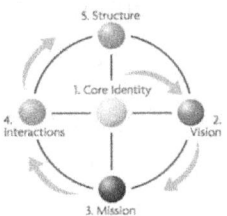

CHANGE =

<u>C</u>enter + <u>H</u>ope + <u>A</u>ct + <u>N</u>avigate + <u>G</u>row + <u>E</u>volve

APPENDIX B:

ABOUT THE AUTHOR

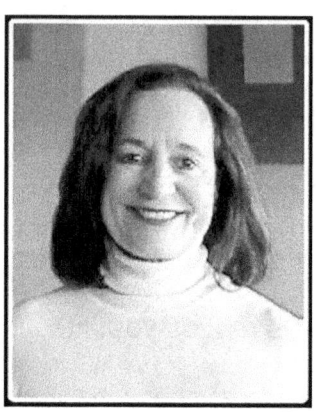

The Day I Learned about Stress

It was on a workday many years ago that I first learned how dangerous stress could be. I was CEO of Central Minnesota Group Health Plan, a staff-model, member-owned HMO--and had just stepped out of my office when I noticed a professor from the local university approaching our medical center's front door. I knew instinctively that something was wrong: even from a distance, I observed that he had a very odd, greyish skin tone that I had never seen before; he also seemed to be walking slowly and somewhat hesitantly.

The doctors and nurses on duty took one look as this patient crossed our threshold. Time stopped for an instant, parting almost visibly between "before" and "after"—and then they leapt like lighting into action to save this middle-aged man who was completely unaware he was having a major heart attack.

Unfortunately, this patient had ignored distress signals and waited much too long before coming in for help. Despite the best efforts of our medical team, the ambulance medics, and the ER staff at our regional hospital, this delay wound up costing him his life. It was CMGHP's first loss, and everyone in our small community—many of whom knew this very likeable, well-respected man—took it very hard.

Shortly thereafter, the entire CMGHP team ramped up its campaign of preventative health care education for all our members; this included teaching the best, cutting-edge stress management tools we could find. In many ways, *SOS: Switch Off Stress* was born in that terrible moment when I stood by, helplessly, as my highly skilled medical team made heroic but unsuccessful efforts to save the life of a good man who had no inkling of the mortal danger he was in.

I hope that this personal story about a pivotal moment in my own life helps you understand why I am so happy to offer *SOS: Switch Off Stress* to help you prevent this silent killer from harming you or anyone you love.

———————

Biography

Sharon Seivert is a business and social entrepreneur who invented *The Balancing Act (TBA)* system—a pragmatic, evolutionary process by which individuals can first improve their own lives, and then help heal their families, workplaces, communities and world. In her capacity as President of The Coreporation, Inc (TCI), Core Learning Services (CLSI), and ThriveSignsGroup (TSG), Sharon has brought TBA's holistic CHANGE approach to people from all walks of life—business leaders, at-risk youth, career-changers, executives, artists, teachers, entrepreneurs, ex-prisoners, and many others.

TCI is a consortium of business consultants, experts, coaches, trainers, therapists, and teachers in the US and Europe. These professionals use *The Balancing Act's* practical tools and cutting-edge methodology to create lasting change for individuals and groups in transition (this includes organizations, business partners, leaders, teams, entrepreneurs, and families). CLSI is TCI's non-profit affiliate. This educational services group delivers career and life skills training to middle school, high school and college students, with an emphasis on at-risk youth. CLSI has also recently launched an educational program for ex-prisoners. Additionally, CLSI trains teachers, guidance counselors, mental health professionals, and caseworkers to use the TBA process. TSG is a technology group that delivers *The Balancing Act's* assessments, interactive guidebooks, and online courses.

Previously Sharon served as an Incorporator and the first CEO of Central Minnesota Group Health Plan; the Vice President of a think-tank; Director of a regional family planning health center; and a manager of political campaigns and initiator of social change efforts.

Sharon's social justice roots were planted early in childhood. Her grandparents were the first "papists" in a small Midwest town with an active Ku Klux Klan. Even two generations later, the anti-Catholic bias lingered in this small community and she was subjected to considerable bullying/harassment. These early experiences of discrimination blossomed into taking action in adulthood for others who were socially marginalized: she headed an anti-poverty family planning center; started a Group Health Plan; organized human rights and anti-war activities; and led public health initiatives (e.g., establishing programs for women's & children's health and safety.)

One of the surprising results of Seivert's executive coaching and leadership work was her discovery that too many people, including those who are considered very successful or wealthy by objective standards, often feel powerless and marginalized—and that therefore, TBA's processes could provide healing tools that worked effectively across the entire socio-economic spectrum.

Sharon hopes individuals and groups use *The Balancing Act's* change strategy to push back against limiting hand-me-down social and cultural scripts that prevent them from realizing *eudaemonic* (purpose-driven) happiness. She encourages all her clients to use TBA to evolve into their best selves. In the TBA step-by-step process they begin by discovering their Core gifts, values, and identity. That foundation helps them move on to thinking more independently, accomplishing their burning desire to do great things, shaping loving and healthy relationships, and then implementing a strategy that will help them prosper financially and in every other possible way. Ideally, TBA's evolutionary process generates a positive personal revolution that benefits these individuals, their communities and the world—to which they can now contribute powerfully, from an abundance of eudaemonic happiness.

In addition to *SOS: Switch Off Stress* (2013 eBook; 2014 print version), Sharon is author of *The Balancing Act: Mastering the 5 Elements of Success in Life, Relationships and Work* (2001 print; 2012 EBook), and *Working from Your Core: Personal and Corporate Wisdom in a World of Change* (1998). Sharon also wrote *The Compass Course* (a 2005-2006 Kellogg Foundation award-winning program for at-risk youth), and co-authored *Knowledge Leadership: The Art and Science of the Knowledge-based Organization* (2005) and *Magic at Work* (1995).

During the past two years, Sharon has worked with TCI Vice President, Fred Reed, to develop cloud-based, interactive guidebooks (IGBs) and on-line courses that are based on the TBA change process and tailored with each individual's

Personal Balance Profile results. The first two of these products, the *Entrepreneur* and *Career Changer* IGBs/online courses have already been released.

In addition to the above, Sharon has written numerous *Balancing Act* web-based assessments and reports in partnership with Fred Reed and Dr. Michael Raphael, an Industrial Psychologist. These include: *the Personal Balance Profile and Personal Balance Preference Scale, Career Changer's Strengths Scale, Starter's Strengths Scale, Leadership Balance Profile* and *Leadership Balance Preference Scale, Team Balance Profile,* and *Organizational Balance Profile.* These assessments and other application-tailored guidebooks, courses, and seminars are available through TCI and its licensed coaches and consultants.

You may join Sharon and other members of *The Balancing Act* community at http://thecoreporation.blogspot.com. You also can contact Sharon directly (sseivert @ thecoreporation.com), connect with her on LinkedIn (linkedin.com/in/sharonseivert/), follow her on Twitter @SharonSeivert, or visit her personal and music website: sharonseivert.com.

APPENDIX C:

CORE RESOURCES

Available to all CORE applications is the foundational book *The Balancing Act* (In both hard copy and e-Book format) and *SOS: Switch Off Stress*. Additionally we offer tailored assessments, Interactive Guidebooks, Courses, private coaching, and certification of coaches and consultants. You can visit the web site of The Coreporation, Inc. (thecoreporation.com) to read testimonials from clients who have benefited from work in the areas noted below, try out several free quizzes, learn more about TBA's intellectual roots, and meet our team members.

Life Balance. Personal Balance Preference Scale, Personal Balance Profile, Life Transition Guidebook, Personal Coaching.

Career Changers. Career Changers Strengths Scale, Personal Balance Profile, Career Changers Guidebook & Course, Career Coaching and seminars. (Upcoming: College Career program.)

Strengthening Relationships. Personal Balance Preference Scale, Personal Balance Profile, Guide to Improving Relationships, plus partner, family or group coaching.

Starting Your Own Business. The Starter's Strengths Scale, Personal Balance Profile, Starter's Interactive Guidebook &/or Course, Entrepreneurial seminars and Coaching.

Leadership Development. Leader Balance Preference Scale, Leadership Balance Profile, Leader Guidebook, Leadership training and Executive Coaching.

Team Building. The Team Balance Profile, Team Building Guidebook, Consulting and trainings.

Organizational Change and Development. Organizational Balance Profile, Organizational Guidebook, Organization consulting and developmental programs.

Below are offerings from TCI's non-profit affiliate, Core Learning Services (learn more at core-learning-services.org):

The Compass Course: A life skills, career preparation and stress reduction program for students and teachers.

The Compass Anti-bullying Program: Addresses and heals the roots of bullying and victimization.

Opportunity Knocking: A career, jobs, life skills and stress reduction program for former prisoners.

APPENDIX D:

SYNOPSIS OF *THE BALANCING ACT*

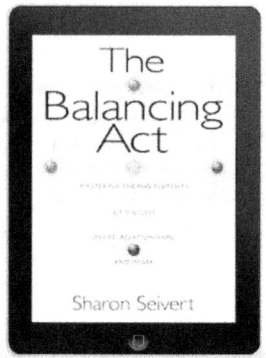

The Balancing Act: Mastering the 5 Elements of Change in Life, Relationships and Work was authored by Sharon Seivert. The hard copy version was published in 2001 and the eBook was released in 2012, both by Inner Traditions, Bear & Co. (The *TBA* print version is also available in Dutch and Spanish.)

Description of The Balancing Act

When the key elements of any living system come into balance, a state of synergy results, where the Whole becomes greater than the sum of the parts. In *The Balancing Act*, business consultant and executive coach Sharon Seivert shows you how to create this exceptional state in your daily life and work. You can use TBA to improve important relationships, lead with confidence and integrity, function better under stress, create wealth, and find the spare time you thought you didn't have.

Drawing on her professional experience consulting in the fields of technology, health care, financial services, human services, and government, Seivert provides concrete examples of individuals and organizations that have achieved positive and permanent changes using her 5 Elements of Success program.

By completing the diagnostic balance sheets in Part I of this book, you can gauge your personal, relationship, and organizational strengths and weaknesses in six key areas:

- *The Core/Soul/Essence:* Core identity, values, gifts.

- *Vision/Mind/Air:* Creativity and inspiration.

- *Mission/Will/Fire:* Initiative and drive.

- *Interactions/Emotions/Water:* Communication & EQ.

- *Structure/Body/Earth:* Practical follow-through.

- *Synergy/Flow/Context:* Connects 5 Elements of Success for balance, wellbeing, ease, and optimal results.

By following Seivert's program step-by-step, you will take a proactive role in bringing your life into a state of balance and harmony. The unique tools in *The Balancing Act* can be applied equally well to businesses, families, or personal relationships.

Each TBA chapter is divided into sections, so you can read only the parts of TBA that most interest you. These sections show how to use TBA's principals in these areas: Personal, Relationships, Leadership, Organization, and the World.

Intellectual Roots:

The intellectual roots of The Balancing Act are highly diverse. They include: the philosophy of American Pragmatism; Systems thinking; Quality/business improvement processes; action learning cycles; the science of *Autopoiesis*, especially biology; modern physics; the archetypal template of the center and four directions; Holistic 5-element healing approaches; Positive psychology; and change management research.

To Read More About TBA or to Order:

To read more about or to order *The Balancing Act*, go to http://balance.thecoreporation.com.

Sample Reviews:

<u>A book with Soul</u>. "I have *The Balancing Act* side-by-side with my *Seven Habits of Highly Effective People*. I find this book to be even more insightful than Mr. Covey's in helping me articulate who I am, what my core beliefs are, and how to balance this with my other elements.... It's like soul music that reaches into your very being."

– Amazon.com customer

The Definitive Book for Life Balance. "Just as Richard Bolles' *What Color is Your Parachute* is the Bible for people in career search, Sharon Seivert's new book, *The Balancing Act*, is the definitive work for those seeking life balance."

– Gerry Garvin, Personal/Life Coach, CPCC

A valuable tool in the therapeutic process. "Sharon Seivert's insightful understanding of the process of emotional growth provides clients with new avenues to deepen their involvement in their own therapy."

– Luisa Bryan, Psy.D.

Illustrates how to create a magical state. "When the key elements of any system come into balance, the whole becomes greater than the sum of the parts. Using highly effective elemental strategies, Seivert illustrates how to create this magical state of affairs in your life, love, family, and work on a daily basis."

-- The New Times

Serves as a Road Map. "*The Balancing Act* . . . serves as a roadmap, reminding me that how I get there is just as important as where I go."

-- Jeremiah White, VP, Fidelity Investments

Brilliant! "Sharon Seivert is a very wise woman who has developed a powerful model that will indeed improve the quality of relationships in your life, your work, and your community. Using Sharon's simple yet not simplistic assessment tools, you will discover where you are out of balance in your life or your organization, and then learn how to create an alignment of the five elements. Her lessons are comprehensive yet practical and clearly defined. If you are ready to change your life, get this book!"

- Gail McMeekin, Author
The 12 Secrets of Highly Creative Women

THE END

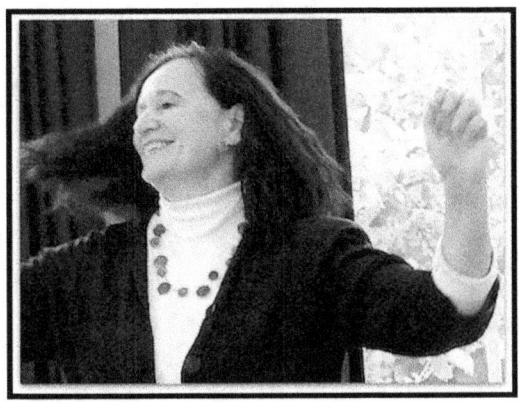

I wish you always,

and in all ways,

the very best of luck Switching Off Stress—

in this moment of choice,

and the next,

and the next.